Integrated Science

Volume 10

Editor-in-Chief

Nima Rezaei ⓘ, Tehran University of Medical Sciences, Tehran, Iran

The **Integrated Science** Series aims to publish the most relevant and novel research in all areas of Formal Sciences, Physical and Chemical Sciences, Biological Sciences, Medical Sciences, and Social Sciences. We are especially focused on the research involving the integration of two of more academic fields offering an innovative view, which is one of the main focuses of Universal Scientific Education and Research Network (USERN), science without borders.

    Integrated Science is committed to upholding the integrity of the scientific record and will follow the Committee on Publication Ethics (COPE) guidelines on how to deal with potential acts of misconduct and correcting the literature.

Stanislaw Stawicki
Editor

Blockchain in Healthcare

From Disruption to Integration

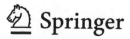 Springer

Editor
Stanislaw Stawicki
Department of Research and Innovation
St. Luke's University Health Network
Bethlehem, PA, USA

ISSN 2662-9461   ISSN 2662-947X   (electronic)
Integrated Science
ISBN 978-3-031-14593-3   ISBN 978-3-031-14591-9   (eBook)
https://doi.org/10.1007/978-3-031-14591-9

This Springer imprint is published by the registered company Springer Nature Switzerland AG
The registered company address is: Gewerbestrasse 11, 6330 Cham, Switzerland

Preface

The blockchain does one thing: It replaces third-party trust with mathematical proof that something happened

—Adam Draper

The modern world is defined by change! Change can take a number of paths, from "slow and gradual" to "abrupt and disruptive." When the latter occurs, associated downstream events can produce a variety of often unpredictable manifestations. Such was the case following the introduction of Blockchain Technology (BCT) a little more than a decade ago.

Initially shrugged off as nothing more than a fad, BCT slowly but steadily grew and developed into a powerful new technological megatrend. The gradual acceptance and an "awakening" of sorts came from the collective realization that an immutable, decentralized ledger can transform many areas where the concept of "mutual trust" is required but not always guaranteed. Examples of this may include permanent and immutable storage of critical information across areas such as banking, professional certification, court records, and real estate ownership, to name only a few. Subsequently, we witnessed BCT increasingly entering more and more areas of our social and economic ecosystem.

Healthcare is among the areas that stand to benefit the most from the adoption of BCT on a broader scale. In a way, BCT implementations are perfectly suited to highly portable, sensitive, patient-specific data that are typically utilized in the modern healthcare environment. In addition, BCT-based systems introduce another key component to the existing paradigm—the true "patient control" of one's own medical/health data, complete with the ability to truly decide who can and who cannot access highly sensitive information that currently is all too readily available to a broad range of stakeholders (often without explicit patient approval). This "patient control" is facilitated by a feature inherent to BCT—the concept of "private key" which is discussed in detail within this book.

Beyond the ability to introduce and ensure much greater privacy and personal control of individual health data, BCT also promises to provide a unique new way to implement real-time medical data processing and medical equipment interoperability leveraging the so-called "Internet-of-Things" (IoT) paradigm. Within the world of IoT, devices can seamlessly communicate and exchange critical data, resulting in an environment that is not only able to instantaneously process large amounts of clinical information, but also leverage this processing power to generate real-time clinical predictions, therapeutic modifications, and create various other adaptive capabilities. Finally, a highly refined data processing infrastructure based on IoT has the potential to reduce medical errors, such as "wrong site/side surgery" or "wrong medication" events.

Blockchain technology also has the potential to transform how critical areas such as medical education and post-graduate certification (and verification) mechanisms function. Here, a permanent, immutable record of one's academic performance, professional qualifications, and any other pertinent skills could be readily accessible without the need for the current, highly cumbersome verification mechanisms and redundant applications. National verification and certification systems could be easily extended across the globe, with much greater portability and translatability across regions, countries, and continents.

Similar paradigms could be extended to permanent recordings of medical implants, vaccines, and other critical data points that currently require the bearer to produce a paper certificate. Seamless access to records pertaining to prosthetic replacements (e.g., artificial joint implants); vascular grafts (e.g., aortic or extremity bypass conduits); or highly sensitive medical devices (e.g., cardiac pacemakers or ventricular assist devices) would provide an added layer of assurance and security to an increasing number of patients who benefit from these modern medical advances.

This book explores the most important aspects and considerations associated with the gradual penetration of blockchain technology into the healthcare ecosystem around the globe. Given the rapid and constant evolution of BCT applications in healthcare, it is hoped that this collection of chapters will provide a much-needed foundational framework upon which further research and discourse can be subsequently constructed.

Bethlehem, USA   Stanislaw Stawicki, MD, MBA, FACS, FAIM

Contents

Introductory Chapter: Early Applications and Evolution of Blockchain Implementations in Medicine

1

Stanislaw P. Stawicki

> *Innovation is seeing what everybody has seen and thinking what nobody has thought*
>
> –Dr. Szent-Györgyi Albert

Abstract

Blockchain (or distributed ledger) technology (BCT) continues to evolve. Since its early debut in the area of cryptographically-secured currencies (e.g., "cryptocurrencies"), BCT has gradually migrated into other economic, governmental, and social spheres. Over the past several years, BCT made significant inroads into the area of healthcare. This evolutional and transformational trend continues, with growing number of BCT applications now including electronic medical records, supply chain logistics, transaction processing (both retail and commercial), academics and research, as well as cross-platform connectivity that leverages the internet-of-things (IoT) approach. There are many other actual and potential applications of BCT in healthcare. This book is dedicated to exploring

S. P. Stawicki (✉)
Department of Surgery, Division of Traumatology and Surgical Critical Care, St. Luke's University Health Network, Bethlehem, PA, USA
e-mail: stawicki.ace@gmail.com

S. P. Stawicki
Department of Research and Innovation, East Wing 2 Research Administration, 801 Ostrum Street, Bethlehem, PA, USA

some of the key developments related to the expanding role of blockchain in our health systems, from established applications to cutting-edge developments taking shape today.

Keywords

Blockchain · Healthcare · Internet-of-Things · Information Technology

In a way, nature is a "biologic consensus mechanism" where various, largely random events lead to often unpredictable or only partly predictable outcomes. Within this chaos and randomness, as the system marches forward, it continues to evolve. For any outcome to occur there needs to be a "consensus" of sorts, where the "circumstances of the event" lead to a unique set of "new circumstances," which we collectively "accept" and describe as "an act of nature." Similarly, the modern society is both tremendously complex and highly structured, yet its very complexity makes any particular event or decision at least "somewhat random" and difficult-to-predict. For example, a leader heading into an administrative meeting may have a pre-conception of what a collective decision of "the team" will be, yet there is a pretty good chance that the meeting will conclude with a plan that may be somewhat different from the leader's original idea. Similar observations can be made about the way our elections, legislatures, and legal systems operate—they evolve, change, and this is all facilitated by "consensus mechanisms" of one sort or another.

Blockchain, in its purest form, is an "immutable ledger" within a "trustless system," where everything happens via a competitive consensus mechanism [1, 2]. Instead of people discussing and agreeing upon "how to proceed," the blockchain operates based on a consensus arrived upon by impartial, highly random, and extremely competitive collection of "nodes" (or essentially a "distributed super-computer"). This "consensus-computing collective" consists of numerous smaller individual computers (e.g., nodes) that work together to build a "51% agreement" amongst themselves, with transacting human stakeholders taking more of a passive role, largely as observers and users of this "distributed information web." This, in a way, makes blockchain quite similar to how both the nature's "evolution" and human "consensus" mechanisms operate—a single participant (e.g., a "node") may not have much control over the overall progress of the blockchain mechanistically, but it can "originate" or "initiate" the discussion that subsequently leads to the collective emergence of a "group agreement" which ultimately drives the overall progress and evolution. This cycle then repeats in perpetuity. As such, blockchain may well be yet another "human-made" manifestation of the nature's and our society's basic "operating system." With that in mind, the current book will be exploring "why and how" blockchain can—and should—become an integral part of the future healthcare system. Once again, the few fundamental commonalities between the various environments described above (e.g., nature, human groups, blockchain) lend themselves perfectly to "consensus-based operations" within highly complex systems, of which healthcare ranks among the "top" in terms of both complexity and the gravity of any system failure(s).

Healthcare is a dynamically evolving, highly complex environment that mirrors in its increasing complexity the growth and demographic changes of the worldwide population [3–6]. In addition, our collective awareness of "what healthcare is and what it isn't" resulted in ever growing number of "moving parts" that can be actively modulated to help improve our understanding of the intricacies and factors required for more optimal implementations of patient care systems, which by proxy are becoming more efficient and increasingly safer than ever before [5, 7]. Parallel to this transformational change in global healthcare, the idea of a distributed ledger did not mature sufficiently to be considered "implementation ready" until only approximately one decade ago. For most participants, one of the earliest and most well-known manifestations of blockchain is Bitcoin—the first and best known cryptocurrency [6, 8]. Of course, other high-tech developments also have come onto the scene during the past two decades, including stereolithography, nanotechnologies, and advanced genetic engineering techniques [9–11], but these advances will not be the focus of this book.

The arrival of blockchain technology (BCT) presented the healthcare industry with an unprecedented opportunity to harness the immense power behind an immutable, distributed ledger capability that can help facilitate tracking, analysis, and data-driven performance/quality improvement paradigms. Never before did we have an opportunity to enjoy the benefits of an impartial record keeper and an arbiter that, when appropriately implemented, provides a unique way of incorporating perpetual quality improvement into our everyday routines and operations. This is especially critical when considering the importance of attaining "zero defect" performance in a healthcare industry that still is far from this ambitious goal [12, 13].

This book is among the first published collections on BCT in healthcare by a major scientific publisher. Individual chapters discuss a broad range of topics, including health information management, healthcare education, safety event tracking, provider credentialing, internet-of-things (IoT), tokenization of both financial and non-financial assets, vaccine passports, and many other content areas. As blockchain-based cryptocurrencies and non-fungible tokens (NFTs) approach mainstream adoption, we are likely to see renewed interest, research and development in BCT across areas as diverse as healthcare, supply chain management, transportation industry, and education. Parallel to the ongoing blockchain research in non-medical applications, it is likely that any discoveries and advances will eventually "trickle down" into other domains, including (and thus directly or indirectly benefitting) healthcare.

Within each major sector of the increasingly global economy, gradual penetration of BCT implementations is creating a highly synergistic environment within which various components working together result in a non-zero sum game. For example, the development of blockchain-based patient safety event tracking will significantly impact other aspects of health information management. At the same time, such tracking will likely require that some of the devices involved incorporate IoT capabilities to seamlessly communicate across the entire system. This, in turn, may lead to interfaces between hospital-based systems and community-based emergency medical service (EMS) systems. And so on and so forth... this regression can truly be infinite!

Although the general perception of BCT by the public is still somewhat cautious, it tends to be positive. As we develop novel use cases and implementations of blockchain in healthcare, we must see to it that the public's trust is not breached and that appropriate boundaries are set to ensure that BCT does not become overly controlling or restrictive, effectively entrapping us within a rigid, indifferent, and totalitarian "information prison" with no hope for escape. Most importantly, it is critical to protect the integral role of human oversight over any highly automated systems (such as IoT) and to preserve the ultimate overriding controlling power in cases of catastrophic system failures (e.g., natural disasters or other *force majeure* events). The latter consideration may be of even more critical importance in the context of the rapidly evolving area of artificial intelligence (AI), which if misused or misdirected could have devastating consequences for the humanity [14–17].

As we look to the future, the growth of BCT implementations within healthcare is likely to result in the emergence of major transformational forces, many of which will be associated with difficult-to-predict downstream consequences. It is our collective responsibility to ensure that any such implementations are constructive, as seamless as possible, and focused on increasing both the efficiency and safety of existing medical delivery platforms.

References

1. Shrier D (2020) Basic blockchain: what it is and how it will transform the way we work and live. Robinson
2. Vidan G, Lehdonvirta V (2019) Mine the gap: Bitcoin and the maintenance of trustlessness. New Media Soc 21(1):42–59
3. Borkowski N, Meese KA (2020) Organizational behavior in health care. Jones & Bartlett Learning
4. Stawicki SP, Firstenberg MS (2017) Introductory chapter: the decades long quest continues toward better, safer healthcare systems. Vignettes Patient Saf 1:1
5. Stawicki SP et al (2019) Introductory chapter: patient safety is the cornerstone of modern healthcare delivery systems. Vignettes Patient Saf 4:1–11
6. Stawicki SP, Firstenberg MS, Papadimos TJ (2018) What's new in academic medicine? Blockchain technology in health-care: bigger, better, fairer, faster, and leaner. Int J Acad Med 4(1):1
7. Zvárová J, Zvára K (2011) e3Health: three main features of modern healthcare. In: E-health systems quality and reliability: models and standards. IGI Global, pp 18–27
8. Bouoiyour J, Selmi R (2016) Bitcoin: a beginning of a new phase. Econ Bull 36(3):1430–1440
9. Kaza A et al (2018) Medical applications of stereolithography: an overview. Int J Acad Med 4(3):252
10. Yadav R et al (2018) Gene editing and genetic engineering approaches for advanced probiotics: a review. Crit Rev Food Sci Nutr 58(10):1735–1746
11. Pramanik PKD et al (2020) Advancing modern healthcare with nanotechnology, nanobiosensors, and internet of nano things: taxonomies, applications, architecture, and challenges. IEEE Access 8:65230–65266
12. Firstenberg MS, Stawicki SP (2018) Vignettes Patient Saf 2. BoD–Books on Demand
13. Gale J, Stawicki SP, Swaroop M (2015) Patient-centered transformation: case clinical examples. In: Fundamentals of patient safety in medicine and surgery, p 142

14. Wetzel RC, Aczon M, Ledbetter DR (2018) Artificial intelligence: an inkling of caution. Pediatr Crit Care Med 19(10):1004–1005
15. Sharma G, Carter A (2017) Artificial intelligence and the pathologist: future frenemies? Arch Pathol Lab Med 141(5):622
16. Scherer MU (2015) Regulating artificial intelligence systems: risks, challenges, competencies, and strategies. Harv J Law Tech 29:353
17. Geis JR et al (2019) Ethics of artificial intelligence in radiology: summary of the joint European and North American multisociety statement. Can Assoc Radiol J 70(4):329–334

Can Blockchain Technology Change Contemporary Medicine as It is Currently Understood?

2

Juan M. Román-Belmonte⊙, Hortensia De la Corte-Rodríguez⊙, and E. Carlos Rodríguez-Merchán⊙

I can't change the direction of the wind, but I can adjust my sails to always reach my destination.

–Jimmy Dean

Abstract

Albeit the best-known use of blockchain technology (BCT) is in the discipline of economics and cryptocurrencies in general, its suitability is broadening to other disciplines, including the biomedical field. The objective of this chapter is to review the role of BCT in medicine. BCT in the health field permits development of a stable and safe information set with which users can act with one another by way of transactions of diverse classes. This context permits the access and operation of clinical information without jeopardizing other sensitive data. Another significant advantage of BCT is that the whole system is decentralized and is conserved by the users themselves; therefore, it is not necessary to trust organizations for depository. The blockchain code is open source and can be utilized, changed and corrected by its users. BCT literature is limited up to date. This chapter narrates the fundamentals of this technology and

J. M. Román-Belmonte
Department of Physical and Rehabilitation Medicine, Cruz Roja San José y Santa Adela University Hospital, Madrid, Spain

H. De la Corte-Rodríguez
Department of Physical and Rehabilitation Medicine, La Paz University Hospital-IdiPaz, Madrid, Spain

E. C. Rodríguez-Merchán (✉)
Department of Orthopedic Surgery, La Paz University Hospital-IdiPaz, Paseo de la Castellana 261, 28046 Madrid, Spain
e-mail: ecrmerchan@hotmail.com

sums up the diverse points in which BCT could transform the epitome of contemporary medicine. The great potentiality of BCT, as its multiple roles in the discipline of health sciences, comprises the spheres of legal medicine, investigation, electronic medical records, medical information analysis (big data), education and the regulation of compensation for medical services. If technological progress persists along these fields, it could result in a radical change in medicine as we understand it.

Keywords

Blockchain technology · Legal medicine · Investigation · Data analysis · Electronic medical record · Education

Introduction

Medicine, like society, is progressively advancing towards a digital and internet-based context. The very principles of medical practice (how medicine is explained, how it is practiced, how it is investigated) are more frequently affected by the utilization of new technologies. Nonetheless, the acceptance of medical breakthroughs has proverbially been slow [1]. In the economic field, the arrival of blockchain technology (BCT) in 2008 resulted in the invention of cryptocurrencies, a genuine drastic change [2].

The inventor of this technology, Satoshi Nakamoto [3], is a figure enshrouded in conundrum whose true identity, or identities, has not been formally verified, albeit he could be an Australian cryptanalyst [4]. Bitcoin is an entirely decentralized digital monetary methodology that functions in an open to the public setting, without the requirement for reliable third-party implication. It is a safe methodology that assures the integrity of the information on which it works. This final peculiarity, most importantly, is the motive why other applications for this technology have emerged and why there has been a dramatic attention in the biomedical discipline. Cryptocurrencies other than bitcoin have also appeared [5]. Some integrate authentic innovations, such as the inclusion of smart contracts [6]. Nonetheless, bitcoin endures the most extensive utilization of BCT [7]. In fact, the utilization of the bitcoin network persists to expand continuously [8].

The aim of this chapter is to carry out a narrative review of the literature on the capacity of the BCT and how it can transform contemporary medicine. In other words, the goal of this chapter is to answer to the following question: Can BCT change contemporary medicine as it is currently understood?

What is Blockchain Technology (BCT)?

BCT is open-source software that permits the production of a big, decentralized and safe public database enclosing organized records set out in a block configuration. A blockchain network is an enormous line of data made up of blocks that are produced over time, with interchanges of data between users (transactions), all of which encompass a public ledger. Users utilize a public key infrastructure (PKI) method that contains two cornerstones: public and private [9]. The private key permits the verification of the user's true identity on the network. The public key includes the address that connects the user to the blockchain's data log. Using the private key you can get one or numerous public keys. However, with the public key you cannot acquire the private key. This is accomplished by means of an asymmetrical cryptographic action based on an elliptic curve. This characteristic makes BCT safe.

Transactions entail the conveyer's public key, the receiver's public key and the value (or information) being sent. This action is carried out within a changeable time frame (10 min in the case of bitcoin), at which time, simultaneously with all the other transactions that have been performed, a new block will be produced. This novel block will in turn be connected to the beforehand written block. This operation shall be replicated consecutively. When six blocks have been produced, that transaction will, for all objectives and aims, be perpetual and invariable. Consequently, each block includes data on all the transactions that have been performed, returning in time to the very starting point of the chain—the so-called genesis block. This feature provides steadiness to the information comprised. Blocks are saved digitally, in nodes, utilizing the laptops of the blockchain network affiliates themselves, who are both users and sustainers of the whole system. The data on all transactions are saved in the nodes.

The blockchain is sustained by a system in which nodes take part, named mining. In mining, nodes contend with each other to find out a mathematical question fabricated by hash technology whose problem is constantly augmenting and whose resolution is attained in a fixed mean time (in the case of bitcoin, in 10 min). The node that resolves it in less time obtains the proof-of-work and is the one that writes the next block of the chain to attain a reward. This same system is utilized by nodes to carry out and authenticate network transactions, obtaining a little payment in return. Accomplishing the proof-of-work needs a big computational effort and high energy usage, which is one factor that confers value to the system.

One of the principal interests of a blockchain certification system is that it is decentralized and preserved by the users themselves, so there is no necessity to trust organizations for storage. However, some shortcomings still need to be improved with respect to accomplishment, latency, bandwidth, safety, misused means, usefulness and versioning [10]. BCT has a number of features that make it very attractive for use in medicine, which are shown in Table 2.1 [11].

Table 2.1 Features of blockchain technology (BCT)

Reliable	It eludes the need for third-party intervention because it is entirely decentralized. Its nature as an open source code means that anyone can revise the code without compromising safety (in fact, this public character is, in itself, a powerful security measure)
Secure	The data contained is encrypted but the dependability of the information can be publicly auditable without access to the information itself. All the information entered is time-stamped and can be traced from their origin through all their changes
Incentivized	The network of nodes needs to be maintained by the users themselves, so an incentive is required. In this case, it could be the incentive of the information itself (the patient would benefit from having their own health record, because he or she could get better clinical assistance)
Differential privacy	The identity of the user can be public without the information it contains being so. The user can define access to several levels of information by diverse actors in the health care process (e.g., physicians from different specialties, researchers)

Applications of Blockchain Technology (BCT) in Medicine

The utilization of cryptocurrencies in the economic field has been a true change. Nevertheless, the utilization of the BCT surpasses that of the merely economic. There is great interest in health sciences in general, and in medicine in particular, for using this new technology to other fields [12, 13]. BCT permits appearance of a stable and safe data set with which users can collaborate via transactions of very distinct kinds. The following are several areas where BCT can help advance today's medicine

Investigation

BCT could facilitate medical research in several ways [14]. BCT could ameliorate the whole investigative pathway not only at the review phase, but also when carrying out the experimental work itself. In this regard, a clinical trial needs a complicated movement of data from numerous protagonists: sick individuals, physicians, statisticians, associations and councils, et cetera. A transaction in BCT needs cryptographic verification, which validates the integrity and veracity of the information, restricting its malicious usage. Each transaction is time-stamped and can be traced. Besides, each user retains a public register of all data and transactions. With the double key method, the existence and integrity of information can be assessed without influencing the privacy of clinical data.

Study Design

The investigation protocol can be saved with all the intricacy it needs, including the statistical analysis design. The protocol determines the kind of investigation, the principal and secondary results, criteria for inclusion and exclusion, end points and sample size. These parameters can be saved and time-stamped to avert it from being modified. This avoids the likelihood of altering the first design based on the information assembled or of modifying the outcomes.

Information Analysis

Data analysis can be carried out automatically, according to the statistical analysis strategy designed in advance [15]. Any try to modify the way parameters are processed would halt the investigation's own code, averting its utilization. This ameliorates information safety and makes the investigation reproducible by another physician. As it is a decentralized methodology and preserved by the users themselves, the course of the research may have to be corroborated by the diverse actors implicated in its execution, which would be a supplemental safety action. Besides, thanks to its capacity to utilize asymmetrical cryptography instruments, it permits for differential privacy. That means that participants can have a share in clinical information without having to share sensitive information. Additionally, physicians other than those implicated in the research could gain access to clinical data prior to analytical processing for secondary analyses, revisions or meta-analyses.

Clinical Trials

In about 10% of clinical trials there are problems associated with reported approbations of research participators, such as lack of consent, inappropriate consent and disappearance of consent [16]. With the utilization of BCT, not only can consent acquiescence be saved, but the research protocol itself can be reserved along with informed consent signed by the participator. In the case of protocol changes, participator reconsent can be reregistered along with the change. This full process would be carried out securely and time-stamped [17]. Moreover, BCT accommodates to diverse digital signature approaches, such as shared signatures and signatures of the same document carried out by numerous users. BCT can also ameliorate the enrollment of participators. It has been published that 80% of participants would be willing to share clinical information if there was a method to protect their privacy [18]. With the utilization of BCT, information can be shared in a decentralized mode, with no necessity for organizations or trusted third parties [19].

Publication of Research Papers

Current scientific publications are based on peer review, which is an excellent system for assessing the quality of scientific articles, but it has some shortcomings. It has been calculated that 80% of reported studies cannot be replicated due to diverse mistakes, in some cases deliberate. Moreover, peer review does not at all times accomplish good control of the scientific excellence of the publication, due to the fact that it is implemented with great irregularity in both theory and practice. This heterogeneity signifies that it cannot be standardized as a system and it is not feasible to know precisely what it signifies that a study is reported in a peer reviewed publication [20–25]. BCT could reinvent the peer review method more effectively, justly and impartially than the contemporary method [26]. The principal advantages of this method are that it is decentralized, distributed, transparent and immutable [27]. A scientific paper based on BCT could set up a method of tokens (counters with no real economic value) as a reward for the diverse actors (e.g., scientists, reviewers, editors), which would be a measure of scientific reputation. Pecuniary remuneration could also be made for the work carried out, acting as a cryptocurrency [10]. In fact, there are already scientific journals based on BCT, such as Ledger, inaugurated in 2015. A scientific paper based on BCT has a number of advantages [26], which are shown in Table 2.2.

Teaching

BCT could ameliorate teaching by enabling the inception of dependable and time-stamped scientific articles and books. BCT permits safe knowledge storing, allowing users to check whether the data they are accessing are accurate. Moreover, BCT allows the evolution of information to accommodate to the novel discoveries of an ever-changing medical science. Based on a chain system, diverse versions of the different documents can be entered to check their evolution. BCT could be

Table 2.2 Features and advantages of a scientific paper based on blockchain

Features	Advantages
Authentication of papers	Averts fraud
Reviewer intervention	Moderates and corrects publications
Integration with rewards	Incentive for reviewers and researchers
Verification of investigations	Eases the replicability of investigations
Differential privacy	Keeps researchers and reviewers anonymous (if desired), while permitting them to be identified as such

utilized to manage academic university degrees and certificates by the users themselves. BCT accommodates optimally to a method of levels such as university degrees, courses or certifications; requirements can be determined to ingress certain grades and corroborate their accomplishment. It can also be utilized to save students' exams and responses safely, encrypting them in the chain itself to provide greater robustness to attaining certain degrees [28].

Electronic Medical Records (EMRs)

The EMR has evolved into the standard for recording, representing and analyzing patient clinical information [29]. The acceptance of this novel standard has produced novel technical (storage, privacy) and ethical (analysis) difficulties. BCT can permit the inception of a patient-centered EMR system. Clinical information could be saved apart from sensitive information, with the grade of specification and compartmentalization sought. It would be the patient himself who could allow the consultation of a part of the information according to his necessities, averting unauthorized entry to the other sections. All information would be saved safely, encrypted and time-stamped, which would avert any undesired modifications. It is stunning how little involvement patients have had in the creation of diverse EMRs [30]. Nevertheless, it has been admitted that most patients wish entry to their clinical information; those who do so are more implicated in their health care. Besides, most physicians and patients who use EMRs are interested in integrating it into their everyday clinical practice [11, 31].

Wise for Meaningful

The notion of judicious utilization has evolved into an important term in health care informatics [32]. The optimum care is not simply accomplished by utilizing EMRs and integrating technology, but by augmenting interoperability and easing clinical decision making during care. It is a concept that implicates all health care professionals, has its exclusive standardized nomenclature (Omaha System) and is based on five essential columns. Table 2.3 shows the goals of judicious utilization. BCT could be contemplated as part of the judicious utilization notion because it is patient-centered and ensures an advantageous, effective and continuous current of

Table 2.3 Goals of meaningful utilization

Ameliorating the quality, security, effectiveness and equity of care
Implicating patients and their families
Ameliorating care coordination
Ameliorating public health
Ensuring privacy and safety

information. This notion is relevant not only in health care practice, but in university education too [33].

Big Data

Another advantage of utilizing BCT as an EMR is that it can be accommodated to be compatible with big data technology. Big data is defined as the storing and analysis of substantial and/or complicated amounts of data through diverse methods, including machine learning [34]. When thinking about EMRs as data, it should be remarked that it has been calculated that more than one billion medical visits per year are anticipated to be documented in the United States exclusively [35, 36]. All these clinical records are contemplated appropriate for analysis utilizing big data methods, which is why an interest has ascended in this kind of technology being applied to the health care area [37]. The development of novel technologies is what is permitting the analysis of huge amounts of data. The enormousness of the data saved not only relates to its amount, but also to the diversity of its data types; thus, the intrinsic difficulty of analyzing such clinical information. In the big data-type analysis, 5 "V" has been reported (Table 2.4) [38]. Big data could be very valuable in a number of fields (Table 2.5) [39, 40]. For some scientists, the inclusion of big data methods into EMRs could fulfill the promises of security and efficacy with which the medical community adopted the implantation of electronic health records [38]. Big data analysis is commonly carried out on distributed databases. Traditional distributed databases are typically superior to those of BCT in their high throughput, inferior latency, superior capacity, rich querying and rich permissioning [41]. Nevertheless, BCT databases have been created to permit the introduction, analysis and exploitation of huge volumes of data compatible with big data analysis [42]. These BCT databases would infer an advantage over commonly held distributed databases. The dissimilarities are summarized in Table 2.6 [41]. These advantages would signify that BCT-based databases could be superior to non-distributed databases, optimizing the utilization of big data.

Table 2.4 The five "Vs" of the big data-type analysis	*Volume*: The huge amount of data and artifacts that emerge in the course of processing
	Velocity: The celerity with which the data contained in these databases changes, which forces real-time processing methods, frequently in an automated way
	Variety: The diverse origins of the data utilized (e.g., text, images, video or audio files)
	Veracity: The necessity to corroborate the veracity of the data attained by processing the data
	Value: The significance of the information attained in patients' health. In this sense, an equation has been reported in which Value = Results + Security + Service / Costs

Table 2.5 Fields in which big data could be very valuable

Ameliorate sensitivity and specificity to recognize specific clinical cases
Ease the formation of cohorts for clinical trials
Acquire population health information
Optimize decision support instruments

Table 2.6 Main advantages of blockchain databases

Decentralized	Maintained by users without the necessity for implication of organizations or third parties
Immutable	Can only be changed voluntarily by the user who has the adequate key, and there is a temporary record of all modifications made (time-stamped)
Compatible with digital goods and crypto systems	Payments can be coordinated in the application itself
Hash chain event structure	Facilitates structuration

Legal Medicine

BCT permits to scrutinize and review any variation in the information, restricting conceivable deceit or falsification [43]. This is paramount in legal medicine to maintain the confidentiality and privacy of such sensitive data as patient clinical information and patient identities [44]. BCT also permits to confirm or strengthen contract negotiation [45] and even ameliorate transplant safety by securely and dependably connecting donor and recipient and all the halfway actions needed to carry out the organ implant itself [46].

Payment for Assistance

BCT could ameliorate health financing systems by refining their entry, enabling multilateral financing instruments, constructing novel markets, approving smart agreements and producing novel forms of compensation for professionals. This could have a deep effect on the patient, institutions and countries themselves [46, 47]. BCT can ameliorate payments between users in different countries, providing faster, more economical and safer ways of compensation than the contemporary systems. BCT's capability to operate on a decentralized basis diminishes dependence on third parties, lessening costs, as in the case of a pilot project to help Syrian refugees, which decreased fees from 1.5% to nearly 0% [48]. Another advantage of BCT is the likelihood of ameliorating entry to numerous levels of clinical data and interrelating them in a stable and time-stamped manner with certain occurrences. This could ameliorate financing, decreasing mistakes and diminishing fraud, which has been calculated to represent a loss of 7.29% of all health expenses [49]. BCT can also ameliorate the management of digital payment rights (DRM). One contemporary obstacle in publishing and entring published data is the elevated fees charged by publishers. BCT could ameliorate this problem by integrating the payment for the service carried out (consultation on a scientific paper, for example) into the entry technology itself [42]. As a matter of fact, some companies have incorporated the utilization of cryptocurrencies as a means of compensation for the DRMs produced, all in a decentralized way and controlled by the users themselves.

Conclusions

The best known utilization of BCT is bitcoin and cryptocurrencies in general. Nevertheless, the utility of BCT goes beyond the economy. BCT permits development of a stable and safe dataset with which users can interact via an ample diversity of transactions. These circumstances permit the access and operation of clinical information without jeopardizing other sensitive information. BCT permits the utilization of smart sontacts, with which contractual circumstances can be set and strengthened via computerized algorithms. The BCT code is open source and can be utilized, changed and reviewed by the users themselves. The great potentiality of BCT, as well as its many applications in the area of health sciences, could constitute an authentic radical change in medicine as we know it.

Conflict of Interest None.

References

1. Christensen MC, Remler D (2009) Information and communications technology in U.S. Health care: Why is adoption so slow and is slower better? J Health Polit Policy Law 34:1011–1034
2. Bohannon J (2016) The Bitcoin busts. Science 351:1144–1146
3. Nakamoto S, Bitcoin A (2018) A peer-to-peer electronic cash system. http://bitcoin.org/bitcoin.pdf. Accessed 14 Jan 2018
4. Greenberg A, Branwen G. Bitcoin's creator Satoshi Nakamoto is probably this unknown Australian genius. WIRED. 8 Dec 2015. https://www.wired.com/2015/12/bitcoins-creator-satoshi-nakamoto-is-probably-this-unknown-australian-genius/
5. Wang S, Vergne JP (2017) Buzz factor or innovation potential: what explains cryptocurrencies' returns? PLoS ONE 12:e0169556
6. Ethereum WG (2014) A secure decentralised generalised transaction ledger. Ethereum Project Yellow Paper. http://www.cryptopapers.net/papers/ethereum-yellowpaper.pdf
7. Coinmarketcap (2016) Crypto-currency market capitalizations. https://coinmarketcap.com/. Accessed 14 Jan 2018
8. Kondor D, Pósfai M, Csabai I, Vattay G (2014) Do the rich get richer? an empirical analysis of the bitcoin transaction network. PLoS ONE 9:e86197
9. Housley R (2004) Public Key Infrastructure (PKI). John Wiley & Sons, Inc. https://doi.org/10.1002/047148296X.tie149
10. Swan M (2015) Blockchain: blueprint for a new economy. O'Reilly Media, Sebastopol, CA. ISBN:978-1-4919-2044-2
11. Cunningham J, Ainsworth J (2017) Enabling patient control of personal electronic health records through distributed ledger technology. Stud Health Technol Inform 245:45–48

12. Yli-Huumo J, Ko D, Choi S, Park S, Smolander K (2016) Where is current research on blockchain technology?-A systematic review. PLoS ONE 11:e0163477
13. Juanma Roman-Belmonte JM, De la Corte-Rodriguez H, Rodriguez-Merchan EC (2018) How blockchain technology can change medicine. Postgrad Med 130:420–427
14. Benchoufi M, Ravaud P (2017) Blockchain technology for improving clinical research quality. Trials 18:335
15. Sandve GK, Nekrutenko A, Taylor J, Hovig E (2013) Ten simple rules for reproducible computational research. PLoS Comput Biol 9:E1003285
16. Barney JR, Antisdel M (2013) Common problems in informed consent. Human Research Protection Program (HRPP). http://your.yale.edu/sites/default/files/commonproblemsininforme dconsent_2013_vf.pptx.
17. Chainscript documentation (2017) Chainscript is developed by a blockchain solutions provider, stratumn SAS. http://Chainscript.Io. Accessed 16 Dec 2017
18. Chu S (2018) Apple watch release news: survey finds 80 percent of US employees would give health data from wearables to employers. iDigitalTimes (2 February). http://www. idigitaltimes.com/apple-watch-release-newssurvey-finds-80-percent-us-employees-wouldgive-health-data-411578. Accessed 8 Jan 2018
19. Buldas A, Kroonmaa A, Laanoja R (2017) Keyless signatures' infrastructure: how to build global distributed hash-trees. https://eprint.iacr.org/2013/834.pdf. Accessed 16 Dec 2017
20. Colhoun HM, McKeigue PM, Davey SG (2003) Problems of reporting genetic associations with complex outcomes. Lancet 361:865–872
21. Ioannidis JP (2003) Genetic associations: false or true? Trends Mol Med 9:135–138
22. Ioannidis JP (2005) Why most published research findings are false. PLoS Med 2:E124
23. D'Andrea R, O'Dwyer JP (2017) Can editors save peer review from peer reviewers? PLoS ONE 12:e0186111
24. Mulligan A, Hall L, Raphael E (2013) Peer review in a changing world: An international study measuring the attitudes of researchers. J Am Soc Inf Sci Tec 64:132–161
25. Bruce R, Chauvin A, Trinquart L, Ravaud P, Boutron I (2016) Impact of interventions to improve the quality of peer review of biomedical journals: a systematic review and meta-analysis. BMC Med 14:85
26. Tennant JP, Dugan JM, Graziotin D, Jacques DC, Waldner F, Mietchen D et al (2017) A multi-disciplinary perspective on emergent and future innovations in peer review. Version 3. F1000Res. 2017 Jul 20. [revised 2017 Jan 1];6:1151. https://doi.org/10.12688/f1000research.12037.3
27. Antonopoulos AM (2014) Mastering bitcoin: unlocking digital cryptocurrencies. "O'Reilly Media, Inc". ISBN:0783324910469
28. Sony global education develops technology using blockchain for open sharing of academic proficiency and progress records. Sony Global, Sony Global Headquarters. 22 Feb 2016. http://www.sony.net/SonyInfo/News/Press/201602/16-0222E/index.html.
29. Blumenthal D, Glaser JP (2007) Information technology comes to medicine. N Engl J Med 356:2527–2534
30. Gagnon MP, Shaw N, Sicotte C, Mathieu L, Leduc Y, Duplantie J et al (2009) Users' perspectives of barriers and facilitators to implementing EHR in Canada: a study protocol. Implement Sci 4:20
31. Delbanco T, Walker J, Bell SK, Darer JD, Elmore JG, Farag N et al (2012) Inviting patients to read their doctors' notes: a quasi-experimental study and a look ahead. Ann Intern Med 157:461–470
32. Martin KS, Monsen KA, Bowles KH (2011) The Omaha system and meaningful use: applications for practice, education, and research. Comput Inform Nurs 29:52–58
33. Martin KS, Bowles KH (2008) Using a standardized language to increase collaboration between research and practice. Nurs Outlook 56:138–139
34. Ward JS, Barker A (2013) Undefined by data: a survey of big data definitions. http://arxiv.org/abs/1309.5821

35. Ross MK, Wei W, Ohno-Machado L (2014) "Big data" and the electronic health record. Yearb Med Inform 9:97–104
36. Hripcsak G, Albers DJ (2013) Correlating electronic health record concepts with healthcare process events. J Am Med Inform Assoc 20:e311–e318
37. Hood L, Flores M (2012) A personal view on systems medicine and the emergence of proactive P4 medicine: predictive, preventive, personalized and participatory. N Biotechnol 29:613–624
38. Peters SG, Buntrock JD (2014) Big data and the electronic health record. J Ambul Care Manag 37:206–210
39. Conway M, Berg RL, Carrell D, Denny JC, Kho AN, Kullo IJ et al (2011) Analyzing the heterogeneity and complexity of electronic health record oriented phenotyping algorithms. AMIA Annu Symp Proc 2011:274–283
40. Kho AN, Pacheco JA, Peissig PL, Rasmussen L, Newton KM, Weston N et al (2011) Electronic medical records for genetic research: results of the emerge consortium. Sci Transl Med 3:79re1
41. McConaghy T, Marques R, Muller A, De Jonghe D, McConaghy T, McMullen G et al (2018) A scalable blockchain database. White paper, BigChainDB, 2016. https://www.bigchaindb.com/whitepaper/bigchaindb-whitepaper.pdf. Accessed 9 Jan 2018
42. Griffey J (2016) Blockchain & Intellectual Property—Internet Librarian 2016. 18 Oct 2016. https://speakerdeck.com/griffey/blockchain-and-intellectual-property-internetlibrarian-2016
43. The great chain of being sure about things. The Economist. 31 Oct 2015. http://www.economist.com/news/briefing/21677228-technology-behind-bitcoin-lets-people-whodo-not-know-or-trust-each-other-build-dependable
44. Szabo N (1997) Formalizing and securing relationships on public networks. First Monday 2 (9)
45. Wikipedia. Accessed 12 Jan 2018. https://en.wikipedia.org/wiki/Smart_contract
46. Till BM, Peters AW, Afshar S, Meara J (2017) From blockchain technology to global health equity: can cryptocurrencies finance universal health coverage? BMJ Glob Health 2:e000570
47. World Health Organization. Declaration of alma-at: International conference on primary health care (1978)
48. Pisa M, Juden M (2013) Blockchain and economic development: Hype vs. reality. Center for global development policy paper 107, 2017. Research Protection Program (HRPP). http://your.yale.edu/sites/default/files/commonproblemsininformedconsent_2013_vf.pptx
49. The financial cost of healthcare fraud (2015) What data from around the world shows. University of Portsmouth, Centre for Count Fraud Studies

The Current State of Healthcare Information Exchange (HIE) and Proposing a Blockchain HIE Infrastructure

Rohith Mohan and Todd Ferris

> *Should you find yourself in a chronically leaking boat, energy devoted to changing vessels is likely to be more productive than energy devoted to patching leaks.*
>
> —Warren Buffett.

Abstract

While there is some Healthcare Information Exchange (HIE) occurring through electronic channels within individual health systems, the quality of information exchanged among healthcare organizations varies widely. The current state of healthcare information exchange has some resource-rich organizations practicing *Modern HIE* with electronic exchange of patient records through established trust among the organizations and technological solutions such as Carequality. These solutions have usually been adopted by larger health organizations but are more difficult to implement at smaller organizations. Unfortunately many smaller organizations resort to *Archaic HIE* as the least common denominator where records are faxed and re-entered manually with diagnostics repeated when a patient's care is transitioned between organizations. Due to its unique ability to decentralize information exchange, blockchain technology could be the ideal technological solution to even the playing field and bring all healthcare systems into the era of *Modern HIE*. Blockchain technology through a novel Secure Hash

R. Mohan (✉)
Cedars-Sinai Medical Center, 8700 Beverly Boulevard, Los Angeles, CA 90048, United States
e-mail: rohith.mohan@cshs.org

T. Ferris
Stanford Medicine, 455 Broadway, Redwood City, CA 94063, United States
e-mail: TFerris@stanfordhealthcare.org

© The Author(s), under exclusive license to Springer Nature Switzerland AG 2023
S. Stawicki (ed.), *Blockchain in Healthcare*, Integrated Science 10,
https://doi.org/10.1007/978-3-031-14591-9_3

Algorithm uses cryptographic signatures and proof of work to establish trust between entities without the need for a third party intermediary. Healthcare institutions can act as miners or nodes in a consortium blockchain to safely and securely exchange patient health information to verify transacted information on the Ethereum blockchain. While there may be lack of interorganizational trust allowing for ubiquitous HIE among healthcare organizations, patient trust in blockchain technology can likely bypass the need for organizational agreement on how to achieve HIE. There are many considerations on what data should be stored on the chain and how often transacted data should be updated on the ledger. Prominent companies and organizations including Deloitte, Accenture and Mayo Clinic have been building HIE systems based on the concepts described in this chapter. Blockchain technology looks promising to solve the problem of health information exchange but much work remains to bring the vision to reality.

Keywords

Healthcare information exchange · Healthcare interoperability · Blockchain in healthcare · FHIR · Fast health interoperability resources · 21st Century Cures Act · 21 CCA · EHR interoperability

Introduction: The Value of Streamlining Health Information Exchange

The modern healthcare environment is complex with patients often receiving care from multiple distinct healthcare providers. While some interconnectedness exists among these providers, health information regularly needs to be exchanged among them to ensure continuity of care. Transfer of information is not seamless and there are often information gaps in which patient health information from prior episodes of care are not available to a new treating physician. Stiell et. al reported at least one information gap in 323 (32.2%) of 1002 emergency department visits, while Cwinn et. al reported that 86% of transfers in the geriatric population have an information gap [1, 2]. Most often, these information gaps comprise of medical history, lab results, vital signs, and medications: all previously collected information which are critical in guiding patient care.

Information gaps affect the delivery of healthcare in a variety of ways. From a healthcare provider perspective, these gaps exist due to the heterogeneous sources of patient health information from different healthcare systems. This forces providers to re-gather this information from new patients entering their system when this data likely exists at a prior location where the patient received care. From a patient perspective, those with information gaps have emergency department stays 1.2 h longer than those without care gaps [2]. The inefficiency of these information gaps adds up from a systemic perspective increasing visit length, likelihood of imaging and additional costs estimated at $1187 per healthcare encounter [3].

Background on Healthcare Information Exchange

The advent and implementation of electronic health records (EHR) was in part to address these issues in streamlining information exchange. While there has been widespread adoption of EHRs in healthcare organizations across the United States due to the passage of the HITECH (Health Information Technology for Economic and Clinical Health) Act of 2009, there is still lack of widespread interoperability among health system [4]. There have been iterations of federal legislation including Stage 3 of Medicare's Meaningful Use Program to further promote health information exchange (HIE), but information gaps remain prevalent due to lack of widespread adoption [5]. Meaningful Use guidelines only provide a minimum bar for these requirements, leading to wide variability among organizations on how these requirements are met. While some organizations have robust HIE within their health systems, information gaps repeatedly arise when attempting to obtain or distribute information outside distinct health systems.

Certain organizations practice some form of *Modern HIE* in which information regarding a patient's clinical care at a healthcare organization can be exchanged electronically among trusted organizations. *Modern HIE* is defined as information exchange of patient data such as clinical documentation, lab results and unstructured patient data electronically. In the subsequent sections we will discuss existing standards for electronic patient data and what *Modern HIE* could look like in the future. The level of sophistication of information shared among organizations varies based on their health information technology (HIT) infrastructure and resources available. Some parts of the U.S including the California Bay Area have robust regional HIE among healthcare institutions built on trust but a standardized national framework for information exchange is still a work in progress. *Archaic HIE* is defined as non-electronic information exchange via fax or paper summaries of care or printed lab records with manual transcription of the records at the receiving facility. As discussed in the preceding section, when providers encounter an information gap even in places that have a robust HIT infrastructure, they often resort to *Archaic HIE* as the least common denominator of record exchange through mediums such as printed summaries of care or faxing records to outside facilities. Some organizations do not have the capabilities for robust *Modern HIE* but in many cases, providers are unaware of how to obtain patient information via electronic channels. According to Everson et al. even when information was electronically queried from an outside organization, providers only used this data 55% of the time given its incomplete nature and cumbersome interface [3]. In the sections to follow, we will discuss existing technological solutions for *Modern HIE* that work in theory but have not been adopted as a national standard. While variability in organization size and resources play a large part in the lack of widespread *Modern HIE,* inability to come to a national consensus on how to adopt *Modern HIE* is an equally big reason why. There are reasons for optimism however as the governing bodies and major players in the interoperability space have an ambitious vision on what they hope to achieve with plans to achieve *Modern HIE* on a national scale. As of April

2021, Micky Tripathi, the recently appointed national coordinator of the Office of the National Coordinator for Health Information Technology (ONC) issued a bold call to action to move all text notes, transcriptions and unstructured medical data to a standardized format through machine learning algorithms and natural language processing by October 2022 [6]. With the recently passed mandate to allow patients to freely obtain their medical record in 2020, the momentum to achieve national *Modern HIE* is at an all-time high.

ONC Vision for Interoperability and Technological Solutions for National Electronic HIE

In 2014, ONC the issued a decade-long plan for achieving interoperability [7]. At the time, the ONC stated that approximately one half of hospitals were able to query information beyond their own organizations and that all 50 states have some form of health information exchange services to support care. They did, however, acknowledge many of the limitations in the daily implementation of HIE and laid out an ambitious agenda for 3-year, 6-year and 10-year goals. By the 3-year mark in 2017, their stated goal was that "individuals and care providers should be able to send, receive, find, and use a basic set of essential health information across the health care continuum". Within a large healthcare system such as an academic center, this has been met to some degree, with information flowing between ambulatory and inpatient settings. However, there is still an inability to uniformly receive and transmit information outside of a distinct health system.

There have been national proposals for a uniform model of *Modern HIE*. In 2008, the Nationwide Health Information Network (NHIN) was established as a framework upon which nationwide interoperability could be built [8]. It was built by establishing trust between private and public entities with 24 enrolled organizations with players such as the Kaiser and the Department of Veterans Affairs. While initially showing promise, the NHIN did not achieve nationwide adoption due to various hurdles in implementation and adoption and likely due to a lack of federal funding as a result from the 2008 Great Recession. The next iteration in a nationwide interoperability framework is Carequality. Carequality is public-private multi-stakeholder collaborative similarly built upon a trust model [9]. There is optimism behind Carequality given that it has had institutional buy-in from most of the major players in the HIE space including Epic and Cerner with many other major players planning to join the collaborative [10]. To date, this information exchange allows for high-level information exchange between the collaborative participants which includes approximately 600,000 physicians with 90 million documents exchanged daily. The ONC has also been working on the Trusted

Exchange Framework and Common Agreement (TEFCA) since 2018 to provide a common set of principles upon or "rules of the road" that all organizations would be required to follow for HIE [11].

While these proposed forms of *Modern HIE* provide some optimism, at the 6-year mark of their vision in 2020, we should have been able to "aggregate and trend information within and across groups of patients based on information from multiple data sources with bi-directional interfaces that enable seamless reporting to public health departments." Currently, there are still vast arrays data stored in EHR repositories and a growing quantity of self-reported or device-generated user data. While the data exists to meet the ONC's 6-year vision, the free exchange of this data is not yet a reality. ONC's 10-year vision takes this one step further and describes a learning health system in which the aggregated data can be harnessed and analyzed for research and provide population health trends.

To bring this vision to life, the ONC recently passed the 21st Century Cures Act (CCA) in 2020 [12]. This legislation mandates that patients should be able to access their medical record at no additional cost and providers choose the technology they wish to use to meet this mandate. The hope is that this legislation will foster innovation in the health technology sector in developing tools to allow a more open flow of information and allow us to continue to move towards the learning health system. Blockchain technology can provide the perfect solution that would allow healthcare information to flow freely and securely between different healthcare institutions, while allowing patients to be the stewards of their own personal health information (PHI).

Existing Standards for Healthcare Information Exchange

CCDs

There have been efforts to standardize clinical data architecture (CDA) in hopes of promoting a more seamless HIE infrastructure. The Continuity of Care Document (CCD) was one iteration of clinical data architecture laid out by HL-7 (Health Level 7) International, the organization responsible for standardizing CDA [13]. The CCD is a summary of care document written in XML (extensible markup language), a familiar format regularly used to encode data that is readable by both human and machines, and can potentially contain pertinent health information such as: allergies, medical problems, procedures, family history, social history, payers, advanced directives, medications, immunizations, medical equipment, vital signs, functional stats, results, encounters, and plan of care [14]. While this was a step in the right direction in providing pertinent health information in a user-friendly and time-sensitive manner, CCDs are limited by the information deemed pertinent by the provider entering the information. They provide only a snapshot of a patient's care, and are often missing key data points or contain disjointed non-pertinent information to the end user. CCDs can be useful in promoting HIE, but only in the context of a patient's complete health record. One commonly used example of CCDs are Epic's *Care Everywhere* which transmits these documents when queried from select outside institutions if the outside institution uses EPIC [15]. However, the fifteen data fields outlined above in CCDs are limited in scope and do not capture the full complexity of patient health data.

Fast Healthcare Interoperability Resources (FHIR) and United States Core Data for Interoperability (USCDI)

Before being able to transfer a patient's complete health record, we need to have a framework in place to define and standardize all the data elements that encompass their health data. To address this need, HL-7 has developed Fast Healthcare Interoperability Resources (FHIR pronounced "fire") [16]. FHIR is an evolving set of data standards that encompasses many more data fields than a CCD and is built on a the widely used RESTful application programming interface (API) [17]. An API is an interface which acts as an intermediary between a user requesting data and the software, which has access to raw data elements stored in a particular location. A user can programmatically request information through an API. APIs are so ubiquitous that we use them daily when accessing webpages. The standard web API used is known as RESTful (representational state transfer). The RESTful API allows users requesting information on different systems to query and obtain the same information stored in data structures across the network. Web based *resources* are documents or files that we access via webpages with a unique address defined in URLs (uniform resource locators). This process of sending and receiving requests is standardized allowing for the interoperable system of the internet as we know it. Requests are sent out through hypertext transfer protocols known as HTTP requests; the websites addresses that we commonly use. Responses are received to these requests returned in an Extensible Markup Language (XML) or JavaScript Object Notation (JSON) format which are then reformatted by an API and presented to us as the webpages we regularly interact with.

FHIR takes this ubiquitous framework used to build the internet to allow the same interoperability and access to health data across different health systems. On the HL-7 FHIR website, there is a continuously evolving resource index with many more data elements than the initial CCD described earlier in this section [18]. Defining and standardizing data elements is the most important first step needed prior to achieving widespread interoperability. Let us look into an example of a FHIR. Resource 8.10 for an episode of care is defined as "An association between a patient and an organization/healthcare provider(s) during which time encounters may occur. The managing organization assumes a level of responsibility for the patient during this time." The data for an episode of care has to be collected and stored in certain format with standardized data elements defined by HL-7, as shown in Figs. 3.1 and 3.2. Just as with the internet, when an API requests information for an episode of care through this resource, the same episode of care will be presented no matter who requests the information. The FHIR library is continuing to grow and

8.10.4 **Resource Content**

| Structure | UML | XML | JSON | Turtle | R3 Diff | All |

Structure

Name	Flags	Card.	Type	Description & Constraints	?
EpisodeOfCare	TU		DomainResource	An association of a Patient with an Organization and Healthcare Provider(s) for a period of time that the Organization assumes some level of responsibility Elements defined in Ancestors: id, meta, implicitRules, language, text, contained, extension, modifierExtension	
identifier		0..*	Identifier	Business Identifier(s) relevant for this EpisodeOfCare	
status	?! Σ	1..1	code	planned | waitlist | active | onhold | finished | cancelled | entered-in-error EpisodeOfCareStatus (Required)	
statusHistory		0..*	BackboneElement	Past list of status codes (the current status may be included to cover the start date of the status)	
status		1..1	code	planned | waitlist | active | onhold | finished | cancelled | entered-in-error EpisodeOfCareStatus (Required)	
period		1..1	Period	Duration the EpisodeOfCare was in the specified status	
type	Σ	0..*	CodeableConcept	Type/class - e.g. specialist referral, disease management Episode of care type (Example)	
diagnosis	Σ	0..*	BackboneElement	The list of diagnosis relevant to this episode of care	
condition	Σ	1..1	Reference(Condition)	Conditions/problems/diagnoses this episode of care is for	
role	Σ	0..1	CodeableConcept	Role that this diagnosis has within the episode of care (e.g. admission, billing, discharge ..) DiagnosisRole (Preferred)	
rank	Σ	0..1	positiveInt	Ranking of the diagnosis (for each role type)	
patient	Σ	1..1	Reference(Patient)	The patient who is the focus of this episode of care	
managingOrganization	Σ	0..1	Reference(Organization)	Organization that assumes care	
period	Σ	0..1	Period	Interval during responsibility is assumed	
referralRequest		0..*	Reference(ServiceRequest)	Originating Referral Request(s)	
careManager		0..1	Reference(Practitioner | PractitionerRole)	Care manager/care coordinator for the patient	
team		0..*	Reference(CareTeam)	Other practitioners facilitating this episode of care	
account		0..*	Reference(Account)	The set of accounts that may be used for billing for this EpisodeOfCare	

Fig. 3.1 Structure of an FHIR Resource: episode of care https://www.hl7.org/fhir/episodeofcare.html

8.10.7 **Search Parameters**

Search parameters for this resource. The common parameters also apply. See Searching for more information about searching in REST, messaging, and services.

Name	Type	Description	Expression	In Common
care-manager	reference	Care manager/care coordinator for the patient	EpisodeOfCare.careManager.where(resolve() is Practitioner) (Practitioner)	
condition	reference	Conditions/problems/diagnoses this episode of care is for	EpisodeOfCare.diagnosis.condition (Condition)	
date	date	The provided date search value falls within the episode of care's period	EpisodeOfCare.period	17 Resources
identifier	token	Business Identifier(s) relevant for this EpisodeOfCare	EpisodeOfCare.identifier	30 Resources
incoming-referral	reference	Incoming Referral Request	EpisodeOfCare.referralRequest (ServiceRequest)	
organization	reference	The organization that has assumed the specific responsibilities of this EpisodeOfCare	EpisodeOfCare.managingOrganization (Organization)	
patient	reference	The patient who is the focus of this episode of care	EpisodeOfCare.patient (Patient)	33 Resources
status	token	The current status of the Episode of Care as provided (does not check the status history collection)	EpisodeOfCare.status	
type	token	Type/class - e.g. specialist referral, disease management	EpisodeOfCare.type	5 Resources

Fig. 3.2 Resource components within the FHIR episode of care https://www.hl7.org/fhir/episodeofcare.html

individual resources are continually improved over time. Resources are assigned a maturity level graded from FMM 0 to 5 as their use and functionality improves over time (Table 3.1) [19].

While FHIR are the standardized data elements themselves, United States Core Data for Interoperability (USCDI) are the more usable standardized set of health data classes used to describe the health information exchanged. While USCDI data elements can be granular like the FHIR data elements above, the USCDI data classes group these data elements into usable categories recognized by patients and providers [20]. The major USCDI classes according to USCDI V1 (version 1)

Table 3.1 FHIR maturity levels of artifacts (FMM)

Draft (0)	The resource or profile (artifact) has been published on the current build. This level is synonymous with *Draft*
FMM 1	PLUS the artifact produces no warnings during the build process and the responsible WG has indicated that they consider the artifact substantially complete and ready for implementation. For resources, profiles and implementation guides, the FHIR Management Group has approved the underlying resource/profile/IG proposal
FMM 2	PLUS the artifact has been tested and successfully supports interoperability among at least three independently developed systems leveraging most of the scope (e.g., at least 80% of the core data elements) using semi-realistic data and scenarios based on at least one of the declared scopes of the artifact. These interoperability results must have been reported to and accepted by the FMG
FMM 3	PLUS + the artifact has been verified by the work group as meeting the Conformance Resource Quality Guidelines; has been subject to a round of formal balloting; has at least 10 distinct implementer comments recorded in the tracker drawn from at least 3 organizations resulting in at least one substantive change
FMM 4	LUS the artifact has been tested across its scope (see below), published in a formal publication (e.g., Trial-Use), and implemented in multiple prototype projects. As well, the responsible work group agrees the artifact is sufficiently stable to require implementer consultation for subsequent non-backward compatible changes
FMM5	The artifact has been published in two formal publication release cycles at FMM1 + (i.e., Trial-Use level) and has been implemented in at least 5 independent production systems in more than one country
Normative	Artifact is stable for widespread use

https://www.hl7.org/fhir/versions.html

include allergies and intolerances, health concerns, procedures, immunizations, clinical notes, laboratory values, medications, vital signs, and patient demographics [21]. These data classes continue to evolve and were recently upgraded to V1 to define clear standards for data element exchange by the 21st CCA. Version 2 is currently being drafted with standards continually being refined.

The implications for this type of standardization of data through FHIR and USCDI are tremendous. Building on the example of RESTful API for the modern-day internet, the ability to create an interoperable network of free flowing FHIR data can move us toward the 10-year ONC vision of the learning health system. The 21st CCA paves the way for the private sector to build applications for health data to be exchanged allowing patients to electronically access their data through an API. HL-7 developed the Argonaut Project to fast track the development of applications based using FHIR [22]. The big players in the health EHR space including EPIC, Cerner, Athenahealth and powerhouse healthcare organizations such as Mayo Clinic and Partners Healthcare have been key contributors to the Argonaut project. The HL-7 Argonaut website details the projects being worked on with a network of applications being developed based on FHIR data known as SMART App Framework [23]. The four main types of applications being developed are standalone patient apps, patient apps that launch from a portal, standalone provider apps, and provider apps that launch from a portal.

As exciting as it is that healthcare data is being standardized and moving towards an internet-like infrastructure, efficient HIE has been stunted by the inability for healthcare organizations to move all players into a standardized form of *Modern HIE* due to a lack of trust and organizational buy-in to a solution unless mandated federally. We have some organizations who have sophisticated forms of data exchange regionally but others who resort to the least common denominator of *Archaic HIE* through exchange of paper records. The passage of the 21st CCA will push organizations to exchange information more freely and will likely facilitate more organizations to adopt some of the *Modern HIE* techniques described above. If we are investing time and resources into this transformation, we should be ambitious and not only bring healthcare information exchange to the modern day state of information exchange, but to the next iteration of information exchange involving decentralized transactions of data. Due to its unique ability to decentralize information exchange without a third party intermediary, blockchain technology could be the ideal solution to even the playing field and bring all healthcare systems into the era of *Modern HIE*. While there may be lack of interorganizational trust allowing for ubiquitous HIE among healthcare organizations, patient trust in blockchain technology can supersede the need for organizational agreement on how to achieve HIE. Blockchain technology could serve as a tremendous vehicle in the implementation of *Modern HIE* as the ONC makes it push for electronic information exchange in the next 18 months.

Blockchain Technology as the Solution for HIE

Blockchain Basics for Healthcare Information Exchange

Blockchain technology is conceptually novel and often intimidates new learners, so in this next section, we will break down the concepts prior to diving into its application for healthcare information exchange. From a data architecture level, a blockchain is a growing chain of blocks connected by a distinct set of parameters. Let us start off with one block. Each block has a unique digital fingerprint called a hash and contains the value of the previous block's hash to connect consecutive blocks of the chain. The most commonly used blockchain hash is the Secure Hash Algorithm (SHA-256) hash, which is 64 characters long and contains the characters A-F and digits 0–9 as possibilities for each character in the hash (Fig. 3.3) [24]. As you can imagine, this creates a huge number of distinct values that could be assigned to different blocks in a blockchain. In a blockchain system there are key rules regarding how the hashes are assigned upon which the whole system is built. The rules are as follows:

Fig. 3.3 Example of a block of healthcare data in an HIE blockchain

Data: • Patient A underwent breast cancer resection at Hospital 234 • X-ray result was transferred from hospital 8923409234 to Hospital 758483 • Lab results from encounter 15959 are provided in the following hyperlink	Block Number 7234 in chain
Previous Hash: 0000HJ2342AS234	Nonce: 567
Current Hash: MB96940CZE1058	

1. A hash algorithm should be unique for a block of data and cannot be used in deciphering the hashes of other blocks of data
2. The algorithm for a particular block must be deterministic and yield the same results each time with the verification being quick and easy to perform
3. Changing one character of data in the block will create a completely new hash identifier for the block of data. This concept is known as the avalanche effect.

The concept of the avalanche effect is the foundation upon which cryptographic mining is built. To add a new block to a chain, the hash value assigned to the data has to fall into a certain target range determined by the algorithm governing the blockchain. The hash algorithm is solved through a trial and error process using brute force computing power. The difficulty of the algorithm is adjusted to standardize the time of interval of new blocks added as more nodes participate on a blockchain. There is a modifiable field in the block of data known as a *nonce* which is continually changed, thereby changing the hash value of the entire block by virtue of the avalanche effect. The particular *nonce* which allows a block to be added to the chain is often referred to as a *golden nonce*. Given the vast array of distinct hash values that exist, determining the *golden nonce* simply requires computing power to guess through the possibilities. Cryptographic mining involves using a vast network of computing power to solve a cryptographic puzzle in order to mine the rewards of adding new data to a blockchain. The value of Bitcoin currency is derived from the *proof of work* required to determine the appropriate hash. Miners who solve the puzzle earn the value of a bitcoin for the energy dedicated for guessing the golden nonce. This puzzle, however, cannot be solved by one server or one computer. Rather, it requires the cooperation of distinct entities, or *nodes*, who all reap the benefits of solving the puzzle. This is known as the *consensus protocol*, with a network of trust built on cryptographic signatures [25].

Now that we have described the rules of creating a block, let us now examine the characteristics of a blockchain. A blockchain serves a ledger of continually added information linked by the cryptographic signatures described above. Each block contains its own unique hash as well as the hash of the previous block thereby linking blocks into a chain. Blocks are continually added to the chain once a consensus of more than 50% of participants in the network agree on a particular hash value. The unique characteristic of this ledger is that a copy of it exists on every *node* in the network. Forging the data on one block of data on one computer in the network would be an impressive feat given the computing power it requires. Corrupting data on the majority of interconnected *nodes* in a network with thousands of copies of that ledger would be near impossible. Given the rapid verification of the signatures and the collective processing power of the network, blocks are constantly added to a blockchain and a copy of the blockchain is being added to the *nodes* of the network. This creates a decentralized distributed peer-to-peer (P2P) network that is secure and nearly impossible to infiltrate [26]. The types of blockchains include:

1. Private Blockchains which are closed off to the general public, with a single authoritative user permitted to document new blocks to the chain.
2. Consortium Blockchains which designate a few users to add to the blockchain.
3. Public blockchains which are completely decentralized without oversight by a single authoritative user.

Healthcare Consortium Blockchain

For the purpose of healthcare information exchange, a consortium blockchain with pre-specified healthcare organizations would likely be the system of choice. Healthcare data is still siloed in individual healthcare organizations, with patients themselves only holding fragments of their own health record. However, over time as the data is freely exchanged among healthcare organizations, a longitudinal health record will exist for each patient even if the organization chooses a different EHR to suit their organizational purpose. Organizations have invested millions of dollars along with years of institutional buy-in for EHR implementation at their respective organizations, so they are unlikely to be willing to uproot their current HIT infrastructure. Given the variety of medical practices in the U.S., there is no one-size-fits-all EHR and that is unlikely to change any time soon. The primary function of a healthcare organization consortium blockchain would be to allow distinct healthcare organizations to trust each other. There would be no third party storing the data and they could trust that a patient's data could go from their organization to another without the data being corrupted in any way. The costs required to put such an infrastructure in place would be miniscule compared to the costs wasted in the current disparate system of HIE described earlier. The importance of the work being put into FHIR and USCDI cannot be understated, since having standardized data elements is vital to allowing this blockchain infrastructure to be fruitful. FHIR, when developed more fully, will allow for the full spectrum of health data to be exchanged rather than relying on simple CCDs. Once data is exchanged on the back end in a secure manner, organizations can choose how to package and present through EHR applications and user interfaces of their choice. Blockchain technology can be built on top of the complex healthcare infrastructure in the U.S. without being disruptive to organizational workflows. Of note, transactional information of healthcare information exchanged would be documented on the chain, but actual patient data would not be stored on the blockchain. While we have discussed HIE at the organizational level, patients are literally and figuratively the key to make this all work.

Patient Keys

In line with the 21st Century Cures Act and ONC vision on interoperability described earlier, patients should still ultimately be the gatekeeper of their personal health data [27]. In a HIE blockchain, patients would need to provide healthcare organizations permission to use their data by linking their PHI to their unique *private key*. This is a well-established concept in the world of cryptocurrency, with blockchain participants utilizing a *public key* to transact on the blockchain and exchange cryptocurrencies [28]. Each user has a *private key* which is kept secret and is unique to each user. This *private key* is only known by the user themselves and is transformed by numerous functions into a frequently modified *public key* which is visible on the blockchain. A verification function can be performed to verify that the *public key* is linked to the *private key* of a designated user without compromising the user identity of the *private key*. While the idea is promising, putting it into practice will be challenging. This *private key* would require the creation of the universal patient identifier, which has been a topic of intense debate for over 20 years. The ONC has long understood its importance but due to privacy concerns and disagreements on implementation, a universal patient identifier has remained elusive in the United States, though it has been rolled out in other countries [29]. As of January 2021, the Patient ID Now coalition is working on standardizing patient identities through improved patient matching and building upon existing frameworks of personal identification [30]. Blockchain's model of using a *public key* to verify a *private key* would address patient privacy concerns maintaining HIPAA (Health Insurance Portability and Accountability Act) compliance in the setting of a distributed ledger of healthcare information transactions [31]. Figure 3.4 provides a visual representation of an HIE consortium blockchain permissioned by patient private keys.

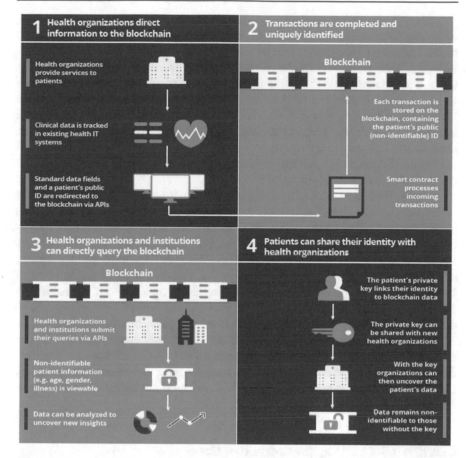

Fig. 3.4 Illustration of Blockchain ecosystem for health data by deloitte https://www2.deloitte. com/us/en/pages/public-sector/articles/blockchain-opportunities-for-health-care.html

Considerations in Constructing a Blockchain Specific to Health Information Exchange

The standard method to establish trust in a blockchain is proof of work as described earlier. In a consortium blockchain where the participating parties are pre-defined, proof of interoperability is an alternative method to establish trust. Peterson et. al describe this concept in which organizations agree upon pre-defined FHIR *profiles* [32]. These *profiles* are pre-defined data standards that are agreed upon by the network of healthcare organizations. If a data element is presented in that specified format, it will then be permitted to be published on the chain without requiring proof of work. This methodology is more human-based rather than algorithmic but may minimize the organizational resources needed for proof of work when trust among entities is already pre-established.

Although standard blockchains are defined by an immutable ledger of hashes, redactable blockchains exist where individual blocks can be redacted by designated users. Redactable blockchains require more effort to maintain but offer more flexibility. If there was abuse of the blockchain with unwanted blocks added to the chain, a redactable blockchain could offer a trapdoor to remove the unwanted block from the chain. Redactable blockchains would also allow the size and scale of a blockchain to be compressed to save on storage over time. In regards to personal health data, if there was ever an erroneous transaction to be recorded on the ledger, there should be a way to remove the erroneous block [33]. The additional time and energy needed to create a redactable blockchain would be well worth the effort in the use case of an HIE blockchain.

An additional consideration of an HIE blockchain is in regard to the frequency of block publication and the frequency of transactional information documented on the chain. The frequency of block generation can be modified by adjusting the difficulty of the SHA-256 algorithm and can be used to maintain regularity as network fluctuates. The ledger itself can be used to document key information transfers among parties but may become cumbersome or cluttered if every single piece of information exchanged was documented. To establish trust between parties, it isn't necessary that every lab value or vital sign exchanged constantly among systems be detailed on the ledger. This issue can be addressed through use of a *state channel*. A *state channel* is when the state of an attribute is updated between participants but not updated on the ledger. You can document exchange of information occurred during a particular episode of care rather than updating the chain with individual events during that episode of care [33]. This maintains scalability and usability of the blockchain.

COVID-19 SMART Health Cards Use Case

A timely use case for decentralized healthcare information exchange would be a framework to verify vaccination status or lab test status for COVID-19. On Github, an online repository of coding solutions, a detailed explanation is provided for the implementation of such using cryptographic signatures to create such a framework [34]. An issuer (such as a lab agency, or healthcare system) generates verifiable credentials which are passed onto a holder (patient or vaccinated individual). The holder then presents this information to a verifier (airline or ticket vendor) who can verify that individual has tested negative or has been vaccinated. On the front end in terms of a user interface, the holder downloads a Health Wallet App on the phone and is asked to save a COVID-19 result or vaccination record from the issuer. A QR code is then generated and scanned at various entry points to ensure verifiable disease-free movement of people at events or during travel. The back end uses a FHIR resource defined for COVID-19 vaccination or COVID-19 test results to transmit information among the parties described above. The cryptographic signatures could be issued if built on a blockchain system as previously described with either proof of work or proof of interoperability between the issuer and verifiers.

Current Work in EHR Interoperability

Given the promise of this technology, there have been many organizations working on HIE through blockchain. Massachusetts Institute of Technology (MIT) is working on a project named Medrec to exchange outpatient and inpatient medication data within the Beth Israel System via a private P2P network and use of blockchain smart contracts on Ethereum [35]. This project is a fascinating proof of concept of what we have described thus far, but definitely requires further research and development prior to being scaled. Accenture has been working on scalability of blockchain technology in order to improve information exchange, as well as assisting patient identity assurance and validation among patients and healthcare providers [36]. Deloitte expansively details their model for HIE with concepts described in this chapter [37]. Their focus includes having a patient key for identity verification and making the technology scalable. They reference the ONC's goals and the need for standardized data formats likely in the form of FHIR in order to develop these conceptual models further. Another cryptoplatform named Tangle developed by IOTA uses a structure similar to blockchain for the purpose of healthcare information exchange. The platform uses a distributed ledger, but uses acyclic graph architecture which may be more well-suited to EHR data. This type of architecture can be more easily updated continually since it is not a continuous chain and can thus minimize redundancy. Tangle also uses a unique method of transaction validation where no parties initially have special validation privileges, but gain more privileges based on the quantity of transactions they perform [38]. This is just a small sample of the work being done and the ideas being poured into this space. There is so much promising work done in this space due to the massive benefits of achieving widespread healthcare interoperability.

Conclusion

We hope that this chapter has provided you with a comprehensive understanding of healthcare interoperability and the promise that blockchain technology holds in improving it. The current state of healthcare information exchange has some resource-rich organizations practicing *Modern HIE* with electronic exchange of patient records through established trust among the organizations and technological solutions such as *Carequality*. These solutions have usually been adopted by larger health organizations but are more difficult to adopt by smaller organizations. The resulting financial costs are immense, culminating in poor patient outcomes due to delays in care.

Due to its unique ability to decentralize information exchange without a third party intermediary, blockchain technology could be the ideal technological solution to even the playing field and bring all healthcare systems into the era of *Modern HIE*. Healthcare institutions can act as miners or nodes in a consortium blockchain to safely and securely exchange patient health information on the Ethereum blockchain ledger. While there may be lack of interorganizational trust allowing for ubiquitous HIE among healthcare organizations, patient trust in blockchain technology can likely bypass the need for organizational agreement on how to achieve HIE. There are many considerations on what data should be stored on the chain and how often transactions should be updated on the ledger. Numerous high power companies and organizations including MIT, Deloitte, Accenture and Mayo Clinic have been building on the concepts described in this chapter. There is still a long way to meet the ONC goals, but there is an urgency to achieve the vision and the technological means exist to make it a reality. Going from fax machines and scribes to a decentralized ledger may seem like a quantum leap, but in regard to healthcare information exchange, replacing the leaky boat makes more sense than patching up the leaks.

Acknowledgements This work was not funded by any institution and solely reflects the works of the corresponding authors.

Abbreviations	
Application Programming Interface	API
Clinical Data Architecture	CDA
Continuity of Care Document	CCD
Electronic Health Records	EHR
Emergency Department	ED
Extensible Markup Language	XML
Fast Healthcare Interoperability Resources	FHIR
Healthcare Information Exchange	HIE
Health Information Technology	HIT
Healthcare Level 7	HL-7
Health Insurance Portability and Accountability Act	HIPAA
Health Information Technology for Economic and Clinical Health	HITECH
JavaScript Object Notation	JSON
Massachusetts Institute of Technology	MIT
Office of the National Coordinator for Health Information Technology	ONC
Peer-to-Peer	P2P
Personal health information	PHI
Representational state transfer	RESTful
Secure Hash Algorithm	SHA256
Trusted Exchange Framework and Common Agreement	TEFCA
Uniform Resource Locators	URL
Veterans Affairs	VA.
Extensible Markup Language	XML

References

1. Stiell A, Forster AJ, Stiell IG, van Walraven C (2003) Prevalence of information gaps in the emergency department and the effect on patient outcomes. CMAJ 169(10):1023–1028
2. Cwinn MA, Forster AJ, Cwinn AA, Hebert G, Calder L, Stiell IG (2009) Prevalence of information gaps for seniors transferred from nursing homes to the emergency department. CJEM 11(5):462–471. https://doi.org/10.1017/s1481803500011660
3. Everson J, Kocher KE, Adler-Milstein J (2017) Health information exchange associated with improved emergency department care through faster accessing of patient information from outside organizations. J Am Med Inform Assoc 24(e1):e103–e110. https://doi.org/10.1093/jamia/ocw116
4. Rosenbaum L (2015) Transitional chaos or enduring harm? The EHR and the disruption of medicine. N Engl J Med 373(17):1585–1588. https://doi.org/10.1056/NEJMp1509961
5. CMS.Gov (2018) Stage 3 program requirements for providers attesting to their state's medicaid promoting interoperability (PI) programs. Retrieved 25 April 25, 2018, from https://www.cms.gov/Regulations-and-Guidance/Legislation/EHRIncentivePrograms/Stage3Medicaid_Require
6. Jason C (2021) ONC leader Tripathi offers tips for interoperability rule success. Retrieved from https://ehrintelligence.com/news/onc-leader-tripathi-offers-tips-for-interoperability-rule-success
7. (2015) ONC maps out plan to improve health it. Am Fam Phys 91(6):354
8. HealthIT.gov (2009) What is the NHIN? Retrieved from https://www.healthit.gov/sites/default/files/what-Is-the-nhin–2.pdf
9. HIMSS (2014) Carequality. Retrieved 2021, from https://www.himss.org/resource-environmental-scan/carequality
10. Carequality Retrieved 2021, from https://carequality.org/members-and-supporters/
11. HealthIT.gov (2020) Trusted exchange framework and common agreement (TEFCA) draft 2
12. Barlas S (2019) HHS proposes steps toward health data interoperability CMS and ONC proposals would implement cures act. P T 44(6):347–349
13. HL-7 (2007) HL7/ASTM implementation guide for CDA® R2–continuity of care document (CCD®) release 1. Retrieved from https://www.hl7.org/implement/standards/product_brief.cfm?product_id=6
14. Lyniate CCD-continuity of care document. Retrieved from https://www.lyniate.com/knowledge-hub/ccd/
15. Epic (2021) Organizations on the care everywhere network. Retrieved from https://www.epic.com/careeverywhere/
16. FHIR (2019) Introducing HL7 FHIR. Retrieved 2020, from https://www.hl7.org/fhir/summary.html
17. FHIR (2019) HL-7 FHIR resource index. Retrieved from https://www.hl7.org/fhir/resourcelist.html
18. FHIR (2020) 2.7.0.2 maturity levels
19. Jaffe CaTM (2016) HL7 argonaut project: one year later. In: HIMSS 16 Conference and Exhibition. Las Vegas
20. HealthIT.gov (2020) Cures act final rule united states core data for interoperability. Retrieved from https://www.healthit.gov/cures/sites/default/files/cures/2020-03/USCDI.pdf
21. HealthIT.gov (2021) United States core data for interoperability (USCDI). Retrieved from https://www.healthit.gov/isa/united-states-core-data-interoperability-uscdi
22. FHIR H The argonaut project: accelerating the next generation of interoperability. Retrieved Feb 2017, from https://www.hl7.org/documentcenter/public/calendarofevents/himss/2017/The%20Argonaut%20Project%20and%20HL7%20FHIR.pdf
23. FHIR H SMART app launch framework. Retrieved Nov 2018, from http://hl7.org/fhir/smart-app-launch/index.html
24. Werkhoven WPTv (2008) On the secure hash algorithm family. In: Cryptography in Context

25. Nakamoto S (2008) Re: bitcoin P2P e-cash paper. Retrieved from https://www.ussc.gov/sites/default/files/pdf/training/annual-national-training-seminar/2018/Emerging_Tech_Bitcoin_Crypto.pdf
26. Buterin V (2017) The meaning of decentralization. Retrieved from https://ictjournal.itri.org.tw/Content/Messagess/contents.aspx?MmmID=654304432061644411&MSID=744064015202124305
27. HealthIT.gov (2020) The ONC cures act final rule. Retrieved from https://www.healthit.gov/cures/sites/default/files/cures/2020-03/TheONCCuresActFinalRule.pdf
28. Reddit (2015) What's the difference between public key and public address? Retrieved from https://www.reddit.com/r/Bitcoin/comments/3filud/whats_the_difference_between_public_key_and/
29. Frieden J (2020) Universal Patient Identifier Needed Now More Than Ever, Experts Say. Retrieved from https://www.medpagetoday.com/practicemanagement/practicemanagement/86865
30. PatientInow.org Patient ID now framework executive summary. pp 2–21. Retrieved from http://patientidnow.org/wp-content/uploads/2021/04/Patient-ID-Now-Framework-Executive-Summary.pdf
31. HHS.gov Your rights under HIPAA. Retrieved 2 Nov 2020, from https://www.hhs.gov/hipaa/for-individuals/guidance-materials-for-consumers/index.html
32. Peterson K, Rammohan D, Pradip K, Kelly B (2017) A blockchain-based approach to health information exchange networks.
33. Nichols PB (2017) Chapter 2: Ideas that bend convention. In: The power of blockchain for healthcare
34. Github (2020) SMART health cards framework. Retrieved from https://healthwallet.cards
35. Lab MM MedRec: a case study for blockchain in healthcare. Retrieved from https://dci.mit.edu/research/blockchain-medical-records
36. Brodersen CK, Leong BC, Mitchell E, Pupo E, Truscott A (2016) Blockchain: securing a new health interoperability experience. Retrieved Aug, 2016, from http://www.truevaluemetrics.org/DBpdfs/Technology/Blockchain/2-49-accenture_onc_blockchain_challenge_response_august8_final.pdf
37. Deloitte (2021) Blockchain: opportunities for health care. A new model for health information exchanges. Retrieved 2021, from https://www2.deloitte.com/us/en/pages/public-sector/articles/blockchain-opportunities-for-health-care.html
38. Using Blockchain to Address Interoperability Concerns in Healthcare. (Nittish Mithal, Mayank Thakur)

An Amalgamation of Blockchain and Connected Health for Combating COVID-19

4

Zhuorui Zhang, Bishenghui Tao, Xuran Li, and Hong-Ning Dai

With COVID-19, we've made it to the life raft. Dry land is far away

—Marc Lipsitch, epidemiologist, in March 2020.

Abstract

The coronavirus disease 2019 (COVID-19) pandemic created an unprecedented stress on healthcare systems around the world. Because critical healthcare resources became severely constrained, especially during the early pandemic, approaches to increase supply chain efficiency took center stage. The concepts of connected health, blockchain, and other related technological advances provided some unique opportunities to address this once-in-a-generation international health security challenge. This chapter focuses on solutions that integrate blockchain and connected health to more effectively address the COVID-19 crisis. An overview of connected health is first presented, followed by an introduction of blockchain technology. Subsequent discussion focuses on the integration of blockchain and connected health (i.e., BeCH) for addressing various aspects and challenges of the COVID-19 pandemic. Specific case studies of BeCH are also presented.

Keywords

Blockchain · Connected health · COVID-19 · International health security · Pandemic · Technology adoption

Z. Zhang · B. Tao · X. Li · H.-N. Dai (✉)
Department of Computer Science , Hong Kong Baptist University, Hong Kong, China
e-mail: hndai@ieee.org

© The Author(s), under exclusive license to Springer Nature Switzerland AG 2023
S. Stawicki (ed.), *Blockchain in Healthcare*, Integrated Science 10,
https://doi.org/10.1007/978-3-031-14591-9_4

Overview

The outbreak of COVID-19 exerts huge pressure to healthcare systems. The advent of connected health, blockchain, and other technologies also bring opportunities to tackle this unprecedented health challenge. In this chapter, we present a solution that integrates blockchain and connected health to address the COVID-19 crisis. We first present an overview of connected health. We then briefly introduce blockchain technology. We next present the integration of blockchain and connected health (namely BeCH) for addressing the outbreak of COVID-19. We finally give several case studies of BeCH.

Connected Health

We have experienced an unprecedented healthcare crisis mainly caused by a coronavirus called SARS-CoV-2 (COVID-19) since the end of 2019. Due to the limitation of healthcare resources in the current healthcare system, making sufficient use of healthcare resources is a critical problem to be solved. One of the promising approaches to this problem is connected health, which focuses on maximizing health-care resources and providing patients with flexible medical services to engage with professional healthcare providers. In connected health, various medical devices and sensors deployed at either patients or ambience (e.g., wards) can collect medical, health, and ambience data via Internet of Medical Things (IoMT) Li et al. [1]. The physiological data of patients can be remotely transmitted to professional health-care providers so that more patients can obtain professional healthcare support or suggestions Syed et al. [2]. The benefits of connected health mainly include reducing the health care costs and improving the convenience of people. In addition, the remote monitoring function of connected health is helpful to reduce the direct contact between patients and healthcare providers, and thus inhibits the infection of infectious diseases such as COVID-19 Dai et al. [3]. In this section, we first present an architecture of connected health and then discuss the technical challenges of connected health.

Architecture of Connected Health

The architecture of connected health is mainly composed of perception layer, communication layer, and healthcare service layer Cao et al. [4], as shown in Fig. 4.1.

Perception Layer
In this layer, the physiological data of patients are collected by a number of connected medical sensor devices. Generally, each medical sensor device is designed for measuring only one particular physiological parameter. The commonly

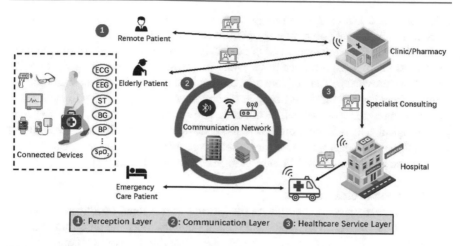

Fig. 4.1 Architecture of connected health

collected physiological parameters include electrocardiograph (ECG), electroencephalogram (EEG), electromyogram (EMG), skin temperature (ST), blood glucose (BG), blood pressure (BP), pulse oximetry (SpO_2) and so on. ECG signals demonstrate the waveform of heart activities while EEG signals are related to brain activity. Meanwhile, EMG signals show the status of muscle's motor units and the ST values are related to the autonomic nervous system. Moreover, the BG values show the glucose concentration in the bloodstream and the BP represents the systolic and diastolic blood pressure of the patient. In addition, the SpO_2 level is related to the arterial oxygen saturation in the blood. These physiological data of patients will be collected by medical sensor devices and then transmit to the communication layer.

The work status of each medical sensor device varies with the diffident types of patients. For example, the medical sensor devices for monitoring the remote patient with mild disease will collect the physiological parameters at given intervals while the medical sensor devices for monitoring emergency-care patients need to collect the physiological parameters with higher frequencies. The collected physiological data from remote patients and elderly people will be sent to a clinic or pharmacy for professional suggestions. Whereas the physiological data from emergency-care patients will be directly sent to the hospital with the lowest delays and the shortest waiting time.

Communication Layer

Most medical sensor devices in the perception layer are limited in size, weight, cost, and computational capabilities, especially for implanted sensor devices. Due to the limited resource of medical sensor devices, the collected physiological data from medical sensor devices need to be transmitted to the communication layer. The low complexity and low energy consumption protocols such as Bluetooth Low Energy, ZigBee and WiFi are commonly adopted in this transmission process.

In addition, the large amount of collected physiological data of patients have to be processed to derive clinically relevant information before being sent to the healthcare providers. The redundancy of received physiological data should be removed and the data analysis needs to be conducted. This process will save much precious time for professional healthcare providers. In addition, the collected physiological data will be stored at storage devices. Due to the large volume of patients' physiological data, in many researches, data processing and data storage are conducted at the powerful cloud platforms Gatouillat et al. [5].

Healthcare Service Layer

In the healthcare service layer, the authenticated professional healthcare providers can access the processed physiological data of patients. With the physiological data of patients, the professional healthcare providers could conduct the pre-determination on the status of patients or even predict the possible diseases on patients.

There are mainly two types of medical institutions to provide diffident types of healthcare services. For remote patients or elderly patients with mild disease, the primary medical institutions such as clinics or pharmacies will provide medical suggestions, while the emergency care patients will be supported by the advanced medical institutions such as hospitals. Once the physiological parameters of an emergency-care patient deviate from the normal values, a special care needs to be done on this patient. Then, both the patient and the healthcare providers will be alerted to take emergency measures.

Challenges of Connected Health

Security and Privacy

In connected health, "security" indicates the protection of health information stored or transmitted electronically while "privacy" concerns the appropriate usage of the individual's sensitive personal health data and prevents the sensitive information from disclosure to third parties. Therefore, it is necessary to protect the transmission and accessing process of collected physiological data of patients.

The cryptographic methods are the most commonly-used approaches to protect the security and privacy of users in the data transmission process. However, a majority of medical sensor devices are small in size, and their computational ability and battery power are limited, especially for the wearable smart devices or devices implanted into the body. It is not practical to apply complicated encryption methods in these sensor devices. Therefore, it is challenging to ensure the security of sensitive physiological data and protect the privacy of patients.

Traceability

According to recent studies Al Huraimel et al. [6]; Kumar et al. [7], there are two main transmission pathways of COVID-19 virus. The first is the direct human-to-human transmission through respiratory droplets from the coughing, sneezing or even breathing of patients. The second is indirect pathway through touching the surface infected by patients. The traceability of patients' physiological data is important in locating the infected patients and preventing the transmissions of the COVID-19 virus. However, the conventional information-sharing methods may lead to the privacy leakage and the patients may lose control of their personal data.

In addition to the traceability of patients' physiological data, the traceability of supply chains of medicines and vaccines is also important since medicines and vaccines play an indispensable role in the control of the COVID-19 epidemic. Many problems arise in the mass production and distribution of injections, such as quality control, transportation, and storage safety. In fact, some suspected adverse reactions after injection have also been found in existing tests and injection results Kaur and Gupta [8]. When any problem occurs, this vaccine-tracing system can quickly trace back and locate the source of the problem.

Briefing of Blockchain Technology

The blockchain is firstly put forward by Nakamoto [9] via the Bitcoin system in 2009. In this decentralized cryptocurrency system, users can deal with each other without any authoritative intermediary's co-ordination. In December 2013, another representative blockchain platform—Ethereum was proposed by Wood et al. [10]. In addition to the built-in algorithms based on digital currency transactions, Ethereum also provides the Turing-complete programming language for the smart contract, which was the first applied to the blockchain.

The data structure of blockchain is quite distinctive. Information is encapsulated into every single block, and the blocks are sequentially combined into a chain. Block cipher is used to ensure that the data cannot be altered and forged. The blockchain system is decentralized and there is no central node in the network of blockchain, through which any two nodes can directly interact with each other. Hence, blockchain networks mostly choose (peer-to-peer) P2P protocol as the network transmission protocol. Consequently, this decentralized architecture is tolerant to faults such as a single point failure.

To be specific with the structure of a typical blockchain, it is a chain-like list, in which each block has a hash pointing to the previous one. A correct chain contains a complete block list and the data. It is available for every node to download and maintain the chain, implying that the blockchain system acts like a distributed public ledger. Figure 4.2 presents an instance of the blockchain structure. Each block in a chain consists of a block body and a block header, with a hash pointer contained in the header pointing to its prior block, which is also called its parent block.

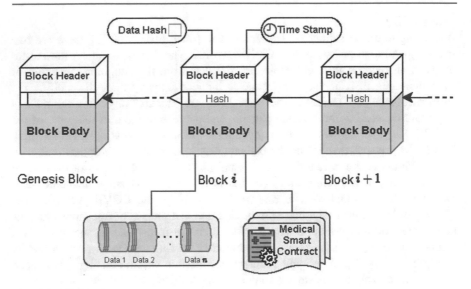

Fig. 4.2 Blockchain structure

It is worth mentioning that the information in the block cannot be modified by others with a hash pointer in the block header. The block body contains validated messages as well as a counter, which could record the number of messages inside the block to guarantee the integrity of block information. Moreover, as mentioned previously, there is no authoritative intermediary in the blockchain system. In other words, a novel mechanism is introduced to preserve the validity and correctness of the information. In assorted cases, various consensus algorithms are deployed to determine how to reach an agreement when verifying and recording new information and blocks. An efficient consensus mechanism needs to allow all participants to reach an agreement in a non-trusted environment and maintain the system under a good fault tolerance. There are different consensus algorithms in different blockchain platforms.

In particular, the Proof of Work (PoW) assumes a race of computing to find a required nonce value to construct the right block [9]. It guarantees a decentralized and public ledger system for trustless entities but suffers from excessive power consumption. Proof of Stake (PoS) can potentially overcome the drawbacks of PoW. It comes from the concept that the more stakes a participant has, the higher chance he/she can fabricate the new block Nguyen and Kim [11]. As an extension of PoS, Delegated proof of stake (DPoS) protocol supports the users who have stakes to vote the delegate or witnesses, to build the blocks and chain, or change the parameters of the network. Furthermore, to protect the system from the attacks of potential malicious nodes, the Practical byzantine fault tolerance (PBFT) Castro et al. [12] despite the failing or incorrect information propagation in the distributed network so as to enable the Byzantine faults tolerance. Moreover, after introducing the idea of voting nodes to record the transactions,delegated byzantine fault tolerance (DBFT) is implemented for saving communication consumption. Meanwhile, Ripple protocol requires less trust to maintain the consensus with low-latency, by utilizing collectively-trusted sub-networks from the larger network Schwartz et al. [13], thereby showing robustness when facing the Byzantine failures.

Smart Contract

As another critical component of the blockchain system, the smart contract is a protocol or a computing program, which is deployed on the blockchain to automatically execute, control, or verify actions under the agreement between different parties. The conception of the smart contract was first proposed by Szabo [14], in order to reduce the requirement of trust, cost of enforcement, and exceptions of malicious attacks during the transaction. On top of the blockchain system, every user can call and interact with smart contracts to conduct various business activities, such as receiving and sending messages, recording ledgers, and voting activities.

Smart contracts share similar characteristics to the blockchain, such as distribution, decentralization, and immutability. Typically, once a smart contract is deployed, no one can modify it, thereby ensuring the security of transactions and system Zheng et al. [15]. For an instance, Ethereum implements smart contracts in various computer languages like Solidity, Serpent, or LLL Wang et al. [16]. When a smart contract is called, it will run immediately in the content of an Ethereum Virtual Machine (EVM) on the decentralized network computers.

In the case of the connected health system, a smart contract could be a patient registration interface, the real-time updating of medical data, or the emergency alarming. Take combating COVID-19 for an example, with an appropriate smart contracts deployment, it is available to achieve the real-time monitoring and early warning of the cases.

Integration of Blockchain and Connected Health

There has been a growing interest in deploying blockchain technology in health-care and connected health because of the benefits of this integration. Blockchain empowered connected health systems can effectively address many challenges and problems, such as the privacy and security of the data transmission, the high maintenance cost, and information integrity of the traditional pharmaceutical management systems. In particular, the blockchain technologies provide more reliable and trustworthy ways of public health data sharing, in which health workers can react more quickly to public health emergency such as the COVID-19 pandemic.

Opportunities of Integrating Blockchain with Connected Health

As mentioned in section "Overview", connected health faces challenges and concerns of security, privacy and heterogeneous of physiological data. The integration of blockchain and connected health brings opportunities to address these concerns. In this section, we discuss the opportunities of exploiting blockchain technologies in connected health in the following aspects.

Security Improvement of Connected Health Systems

While connected health provides patients with additional flexibility by allowing them to obtain professional services and suggestions from healthcare providers remotely, the leakage of patients' information can pose serious threats to patients. Unfortunately, due to the limited resources such as the computing ability, memory and energy power of most medical sensor devices, it is not applicable to deploy complicated encryption schemes in these devices. During the process of patients' sensitive physiological information transmission, the data from medical sensor devices, data gateways to server devices can be illegally wiretapped. To ensure the security of patients' sensitive physiological data, researchers in Zhai et al. [17] proposed an advanced encryption standard algorithm and an ECG identification system while the work of Lin et al. [18] proposed a differential privacy protection model to produce enough interference to data, thereby preventing from matching a certain patient by analyzing the ECG data.

However, the sensitive physiological big data remains being managed by the third party, which puts both patients and healthcare providers at the risk of mistakenly or intentionally data releasing caused by bugs on data servers. To tackle these concerns, integrating connected health systems with block chain is a potential solution to improve the security. Meanwhile, this solution is not constrained by the limited resources of medical sensor devices.

First, the built-in algorithms (e.g., asymmetric encryption/decryption and the digital signature) of blockchain make the patients' data difficult to be tampered. Second, instead of relying on a central authority of control, blockchain uses consensus protocols to validate transactions and store data. The decentralized and distributed ledgers of blockchain reduce the system failures caused by a single point of failure. Third, the firmware of medical sensor devices can be upgraded automatically by embedding smart contracts in them.

Privacy Protection of Connected Health Data

Compared with traditional centralized servers, as a decentralized, anonymous and tamper-proof distributed ledger technology, blockchain provides a new approach to ensure the privacy preservation in medical service. Medical data leakage can be divided into non-interactive leakage and interactive leakage. Non-interactive leakage refers to the leakage caused by internal systems or personnel activities, such as selling or abusing private information. Interactive leakage refers to the leakage of medical information when it is released and shared among different institutions.

Due to the significant value of patients' physiological information, the central node in centralized information system has the motivation to disclose privacy. Meanwhile, the medical data storage depends on the hospital information departments, which lack of security defense capability and technical measures.

To address the privacy leakage in connected health systems, blockchain technologies have advantages compared to centralized servers in following aspects. First, as a type of peer-to-peer network, it is difficult to wiretap blockchain information. Blockchain nodes communicate through a relay-forwarding method, therefore the traditional method of eavesdropping on network traffic to find the relationship between users is not applicable, making it challenging for attackers to find the real source and destination of the medical information. Second, blockchain can hide the account addresses. The address in the blockchain is generated by the user's public key and is not associated with the user's identity information. The addresses therefore can be used as the user's pseudonym in the blockchain system. Third, in the decentralized architecture, it do not require to store sensitive data on central servers, which can avoid the risk of privacy leakage caused by traditional server attacks.

Traceability of Connected Health Data
In blockchain-empowered connected health (BeCH) systems, patients' physiological data can be stored in on-blockchain or off-blockchain manners. Thanks to the consensus mechanisms and asymmetric cryptographic schemes of blockchain, the on-blockchain data is essentially traceable in the whole connected health system.

However, for some data with massive volumes such as high-resolution images and videos, it is unrealistic to store them all on-blockchain. In this context, these massive data can be stored in the off-blockchain manner and we may only store their meta-data or hash values at blockchain to save the storage cost and improve their traceability. In addition to make data traceable, the blockchain-empowered connected health systems also show potential in establishing traceable supply chains of medicines and vaccines to maintain the reasonable production and distribution of critical medicines. Moreover, the technologies of IoMT also propel the development of connected health systems especially in connecting intelligent sensors, devices, software and networks. Armed with medical sensor devices, Quick Response (QR) tags, and Radio-frequency identification (RFID) tags in IoMT, the traceability and immutability of medicines in BeCH systems can be further improved.

Architecture of Blockchain-Empowered Connected Health

The integration of blockchain and connected health systems has shown potentials in improving the security, privacy,and trace ability of the whole system. The architecture of this integrating system namely Blockchain-empowered Connected Health (BeCH) is shown in Fig. 4.3. In particular, we divide the whole system into four

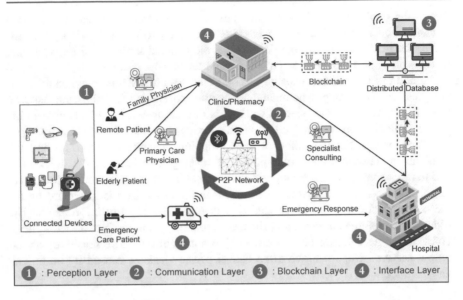

Fig. 4.3 Architecture of BeCH

layers: (1) perception layer, (2) communication layer, (3) blockchain layer, (4) interface layer.

The perception layer consists of connected medical sensor devices (e.g., wristband sensors and blood pressure sensors) and other medical supplies such as medicines that can be obtained from local clinics, pharmacies or online retailers. According to the different demands and conditions of various patients, we roughly categorize patients into three types: remote patients, independent elderly patients, and emergency care patients.

In the communication layer, we can exploit different wireless networking protocols or schemes (e.g., Bluetooth, WiFi and 5G) to facilitate the communication between smart devices. Moreover, patients' sensitive physiological data is stored in a distributed database based on various smart devices from patients and medical service providers. We therefore model this network of communication as a P2P network in the communication layer.

In the blockchain layer, the blockchain technologies bridge different layers as a middleware. Being endowed with blockchain technologies including cryptographic algorithms, consensus mechanisms, P2P network and smart contracts, this layer serves for the entire BeCH system in aspects of protecting data security and privacy, data storage, data sharing, effective authentication and access control.

The interface layer enables different service providers or applications communicate efficiently and make collaborative decisions. For instance, local clinics and pharmacies may have to connect with specialist from remote hospitals to obtain professional instructions. The physiological data collected by medical sensors also needs patients' digital signature before being submitted to medical services. To ensure the data security, services need to verify the signature after receiving the data. In this layer, we can also deploy medical data analytic applications to help analyze patients' health condition and promote a more rational approach to patient care based on artificial intelligence, machine learning and deep learning algorithms. By integrating the connected health systems with blockchain technologies, health-related data such as physiological data and reasonable diagnosis suggestions can communicate securely in real time.

Case Study

In this section, we elaborate the application of BeCH systems on combating COVID-19 pandemic to enhance the healthcare in different areas impacted by this outbreak. The use-cases of BeCH are given as follows: (1) prevention of infectious diseases, (2) clinical trail management, (3) traceable medical supply chain.

Prevention of Infectious Diseases

As illustrated in Fig. 4.4, keeping safe social distance and sufficient ventilation is an effective countermeasure to control infectious diseases including the COVID-19 pandemic Sun and Zhai [19]. Blockchain-empowered connected health systems can provide solutions of quarantine and social distancing. For patients with mild diseases in remote and rural area, BeCH systems reduce the necessity of a long-distance traveling to major hospitals. Supported by the real-time health monitoring of connected medical sensors and remote diagnosis, we can reduce the population mobility, the cross infections and the stress of overcrowded hospitals during outbreaks of infectious diseases. Being different from traditional healthcare systems that are managed by centralized authorities, the distributed ledger and P2P network of blockchain can overcome the risk of single-point failures. Moreover, the main benefits of adopting BeCH systems in remote healthcare include: (1) helping to establish immutable and trustworthy electronic medical records with well integrity; (2) access controlling of patients' sensitive information; (3) allowing safe and automatic micro-payments for remote healthcare services Ahmad et al. [20]; Azim et al. 21].

During the outbreak of contagious diseases, the quarantine for a large number of inbound passengers is a necessary but challenging task. For example, many healthcare institutions were overloaded with receiving massive passengers during the on-going COVID-19 pandemic. In this context, BeCH systems provide solutions of reliable home or hotel quarantines. For example, we can adopt the IoMT in a BeCH system and require passengers to wear a smart bracelet which collects the information of their location and temperature and sends the data to disease control sectors, as shown in Fig. 4.4. The blockchain-empowered connected health system can also monitor people's social distance and give warnings for overcrowded people.

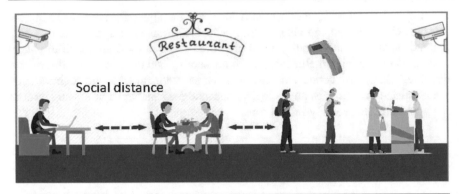

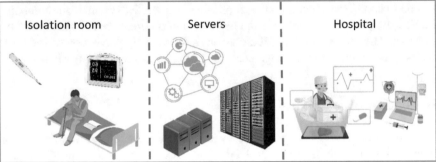

Fig. 4.4 Prevention of infectious diseases

Clinical Trial Management

Before we bring new medicines and medical devices to the general public, the rigorous, thorough and systematic clinical trials and testing should be conducted to ensure the safety and disclose possible adverse reactions. There are commonly four stages in a clinical trail, in which the third Phase requires a large number of participants and volunteers. However, traditional clinical trial management systems lack of ability to operate efficiently while facing the heavy time costs and resource-demanding. In each stage of a clinical trial, helathcare sectors have to collect prodigious amounts of information. Moreover, clinical protocols are expected to have cost-effectiveness, regulatory compliance, auditability, safety, fastness, and transparency. To tackle these concerns, by enabling researchers to upload and record clinical data in real time, BeCH systems can improve the security, sharing and traceability of clinical data as well as accelerating the trail process Nugent et al. [22].

As shown in Fig. 4.5, the blockchain technology in our BeCH system can address the challenges in traditional clinical trial data management by constructing a more transparent and secure data sharing between multi clinical sites and remote participants such as Data Safety and Monitoring Board (DSMB), Institutional

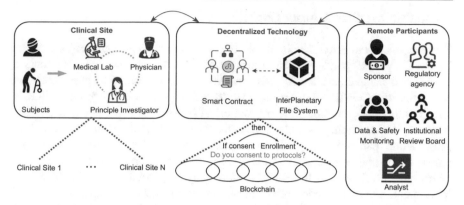

Fig. 4.5 Clinical trial management

Review Board (IRB) and analysts. In Fig. 4.5, we divide the stakeholders in clinical trial management systems into two types: (1) multi clinical sites and (2) remote participants. In each clinical site, researchers (e.g., physicians and principle investigators) collect the data of subjects and conduct clinical trails. Regarding the remote participants, the sponsors are from individuals or institutions who manage and fund the clinical trails. In particular, monitoring boards and agencies such as the Food and Drug Administration (FDA), DSMB and IRB are responsible for evaluating the research data, protecting the rights and safety, conducting ethical reviews and making recommendations Marcus et al. [23]. To decentralize data management in clinical trials and enhance the communication between clinical sites and remote participants, we can incorporate the smart contracts in BeCH systems with Inter-Planetary system (IPFS) networks to store hashed files on the blockchain. By giving a unique cryptographic hash for each file, we are able to track and retrieve these files at anytime Omar et al. [24]. In particular, documents such as Investigational New Drug (IND) application, Case Report Forms (CRFs) and Adverse Event (SAE) are applicable to be stored on the IPFS. Moreover, this system helps to improve the transparency and traceability of the developing and revising the clinical trial consent for protocols Benchoufi and Ravaud [25].

In Benchoufi and Ravaud [25], researchers investigated the significant opportunities blockchain provides for clinical research: defined a set of core metadata, it can examine the integrity of clinical trials transparently. In addition to storing compilable clinical research metadata at each phase, the smart contract of blockchain aids researchers to slice and chain distinct clinical trial steps in order to enhance the stage transparency, traceability and the entire clinical research process management. In BeCH systems, connected health allow researchers and patient communities contact globally and closely, researchers also can collect and share the IoMT data flow with characteristics of individual granularity, decentralization and safety by integrating connected health with blockchain technologies.

Traceable Medical Supply Chain

The world has witnessed the significant medical supply chain interruptions caused by the COVID-19 pandemic. The shortage of medical supplies such as vaccines, masks, and nucleic acid testing kits presents severe hardships to preventing and combating the COVID-19 epidemic. Due to the imposed lockdown and failure to satisfy safe work conditions, the production of factories is at a standstill. Besides, importing and exporting bans also impact the worldwide medical supply Kalla et al. [26]. While panic-buying leads to further crises in supply and demand, the unreasonable and non-transparent distribution is serious problems that need to be addressed. In this aspect, the BeCH system plays a pivotal role in establishing a transparent, secure, and traceable medical supply chain. For example, using RFID tags, QR, Bar code tags, and medical sensors on products can effectively encapsulate the information on the supply chain, such as sources of products, Logistics information, and regional medicines distribution. Moreover, to reduce the risk of infection, contact-lessdelivery of medicines is necessary, especially in high COVID-19-transmission regions. In this case, we can adopt unmanned aerial vehicle (UAV) transportation to deliver medicines and household essentials to remote patients based on the BeCH system. In particular, with online assistant and guidance from medical staff, the general public may be able to conduct nucleic acid self-testing at home while Nucleic Acid Detection Kits are delivered by UAVs (Fig. 4.6).

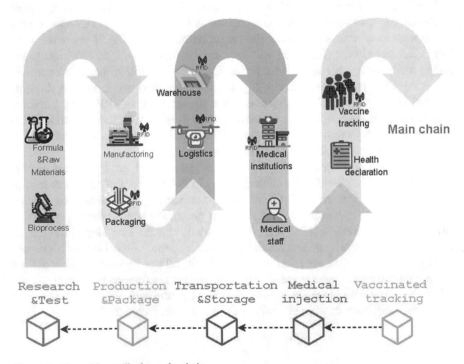

Fig. 4.6 Traceable medical supply chain

Precisely, a traceable medical supply chain consists of the following parts: research and test, production and package, transportation and storage, medical injection, and vaccinated tracking. The data records of each stage will be encapsulated into the corresponding block. Due to the blockchain system's immutability and data integrity, the connected health data will be appropriately recorded and stored and can be traced anytime and anywhere.

Summary

Under the vital need to combat the COVID-19, we first present the architecture of blockchain-empowered connected health systems (BeCH). When facing the typical challenges of traditional medical data management, this novel design is of potential in improving security, privacy, and traceability.

This chapter presented a brief overview of connected health, blockchain technologies and introduced our BeCH system framework. In the design of BeCH, the system includes four layers: perception layer, communication layer, blockchain layer, and interface layer. We also discussed its applicability and use cases of BeCH, such as Prevention of infectious diseases, Clinical trial management, and Traceable medical supply chain. For future work, we believe the amalgamation of blockchain and connected health can bring up more brilliant insights for combating COVID-19.

References

1. Li X, Dai H-N, Wang Q, Imran M, Li D, Imran MA (2020) Securing internet of medical things with friendly-jamming schemes. Comp Commun 160:431–442. ISSN 01403664. https://doi.org/10.1016/j.comcom.2020.06.026. https://www.sciencedirect.com/science/article/pii/S0140366420310227
2. Syed L, Jabeen S, Manimala S, Alsaeedi A (2019) Smart healthcare framework for ambient assisted living using iomt and big data analytics techniques. Futur Gener Comput Syst 101:136–151
3. Dai HN, Imran M, Haider N (2020) Blockchain-enabled internet of medical things to combat covid-19. IEEE Internet Things Magaz 3(3):52–57. https://doi.org/10.1109/IOTM.0001.2000087
4. Cao R, Tang Z, Liu C, Veeravalli B (2020) A scalable multicloud storage architecture for cloud-supported medical internet of things. IEEE Internet Things J 7(3):1641–1654
5. Gatouillat A, Badr Y, Massot B, Sejdić E (2018) Internet of medical things: a review of recent contributions dealing with cyber-physical systems in medicine. IEEE Internet Things J 5 (5):3810–3822
6. Al Huraimel K, Alhosani M, Kunhabdulla S, Stietiya MH (2020) Sars-cov-2 in the environment: modes of transmission, early detection and potential role of pollutions. Sci Total Environ 744:140946
7. Kumar M, Taki K, Gahlot R, Sharma A, Dhangar K (2020) A chronicle of sars-cov-2: Part-i - epidemiology, diagnosis, prognosis, transmission and treatment. Sci Total Environ 734:139278

8. Kaur SP, Gupta V (2020) COVID-19 vaccine: a comprehensive status report. Virus Res 288:198114. ISSN 0168–1702. https://doi.org/10.1016/j.virusres.2020.198114. http://www.sciencedirect.com/science/article/pii/S0168170220310212

9. Nakamoto S (2019) Bitcoin: a peer-to-peer electronic cash system. Technical report, Manubot

10. Wood G et al (2014) Ethereum: a secure decentralised generalised transaction ledger. Ethereum Project Yellow Paper 151(2014):1–32

11. Nguyen G-T, Kim K (2018) A survey about consensus algorithms used in blockchain. J Inform Process Syst 14(1)

12. Castro M, Liskov B, et al (1999) Practical byzantine fault tolerance. OSDI 99:173–186

13. Schwartz D, Youngs N, Britto A, et al (2014) The ripple protocol consensus algorithm. Ripple Labs Inc White Paper 5(8)

14. Szabo N (1996) Smart contracts: building blocks for digital markets. EXTROPY J Transhuman Thought,(16) 18(2)

15. Zheng Z, Xie S, Dai HN, Chen W, Chen X, Weng J, Imran M (2020) An overview on smart contracts: challenges, advances and platforms. Fut Generat Comp Syst 105:475–491. ISSN 0167–739X. https://doi.org/10.1016/j.future.2019.12.019. https://www.sciencedirect.com/science/article/pii/S0167739X19316280

16. Wang S, Yuan Y, Wang X, Li J, Qin R, Wang FY (2018) An overview of smart contract: architecture, applications, and future trends. In: 2018 IEEE intelligent vehicles symposium (IV). IEEE, pp 108–113

17. Zhai X, Ali AAS, Amira A, Bensaali F (2017) Ecg encryption and identification based security solution on the zynq soc for connected health systems. J Parallel Distrib Comp 106:143–152

18. Lin C, Song Z, Song H, Zhou Y, Wang Y, Guowei W (2016) Differential privacy preserving in big data analytics for connected health. J Med Syst 40(4):97

19. Sun C, Zhai Z (2020) The efficacy of social distance and ventilation effectiveness in preventing covid-19 transmission. Sustain Cities Soc 62:102390. ISSN 2210–6707. https://doi.org/10.1016/j.scs.2020.102390. http://www.sciencedirect.com/science/article/pii/S2210670720306119

20. Ahmad RW, Salah K, Jayaraman R, Yaqoob I, Ellahham S, Omar M (2020) Blockchain and covid-19 pandemic: applications and challenges

21. Azim A, Islam MN, Spranger PE (2020) Blockchain and novel coronavirus: Towards preventing covid-19 and future pandemics. Iberoamerican J Med 2(3):215–218

22. Nugent T, Upton D, Cimpoesu M (2016) Improving data transparency in clinical trials using blockchain smart contracts. F1000Research 5:2541. doi: https://doi.org/10.12688/f1000research.9756.1

23. Marcus CL, Moore RH, Rosen CL, Giordani B, Garetz SL, Taylor HG, Redline S (2014) A randomized trial of adenotonsillectomy for childhood sleep apnea. Surv Anesthesiol 58:41. https://doi.org/10.1097/01.SA.0000441005.88110.fc

24. Omar IA, Jayaraman R, Salah K, Simsekler MCE, Yaqoob I, Ellahham S (2020) Ensuring protocol compliance and data transparency in clinical trials using blockchain smart contracts. BMC Med Res Methodol 20

25. Benchoufi M, Ravaud P (2017) Block chain technology for improving clinical research quality. Trials 18:12. https://doi.org/10.1186/s13063-017-2035-z

26. Kalla A, Hewa T, Mishra RA, Ylianttila M, Liyanage M (2020) The role of blockchain to fight against covid-19. IEEE Eng Manage Rev 48(3):85–96. https://doi.org/10.1109/EMR.2020.3014052

Applications of Blockchain Technology in the COVID-19 Era

5

Juan M. Roman-Belmonte⊙, Hortensia De la Corte-Rodriguez⊙, and E. Carlos Rodriguez-Merchan⊙

> *Often when you think you're at the end of something, you're at the beginning of something else.*
>
> –Fred Rodgers

Abstract

On March 11, 2020 the WHO declared a global pandemic state and the virus is currently accountable for millions of infections and hundreds of thousands of deceases. The pandemic has aggravated the crisis of confidence in many health organizations and government institutions, and has generated a number of needs. New technologies can be used to meet these needs and mitigate some of the problems associated with the pandemic. Blockchain technology (BCT) is characterized by being decentralized, safe, independent of trusted third parties and maintaining the privacy of the information it stores, which has augmented its interest in times of pandemic. From an epidemiological point of view, it can help to rapidly detect the sources of infection, processing the information by individuals, institutions and governments. In addition, it permits data to be collected efficiently by ensuring its origin, storing the information immutably and making an auditable and traceable record over time of any modifications to the data. Furthermore, it is ideal for facilitating the traceability of supply chains,

J. M. Roman-Belmonte
Department of Physical and Rehabilitation Medicine, Cruz Roja San José y Santa Adela University Hospital, Madrid, Spain

H. De la Corte-Rodriguez
Department of Physical and Rehabilitation Medicine, La Paz University Hospital-IdiPaz, Madrid, Spain

E. C. Rodriguez-Merchan (✉)
Department of Orthopedic Surgery, La Paz University Hospital-IdiPaz,
Paseo de la Castellana 261, 28046 Madrid, Spain
e-mail: ecrmerchan@hotmail.com

© The Author(s), under exclusive license to Springer Nature Switzerland AG 2023
S. Stawicki (ed.), *Blockchain in Healthcare*, Integrated Science 10,
https://doi.org/10.1007/978-3-031-14591-9_5

calculating inventory, and being able to establish an appropriate balance between suppliers and consumers. On the other hand, BCT could ameliorate the whole process of data processing necessary in scientific research, since it generates a distributed ledger that guarantees the immutability, transparency and traceability of the data even between two or more distant parties with no mutual trust. New working models, access to intelligent contracts and financing circuits, can also be ameliorated with BCT, helping to reduce mistakes and diminish fraud.

Keywords

Blockchain technology · COVID-19 · Applications

Introduction

Severe acute respiratory syndrome coronavirus-2 (SARS-CoV2), known as COVID-19, is a novel coronavirus that became known in December 2019 in the Wuhan region of China [1]. On March 11, 2020, the World Health Organization (WHO) declared a global pandemic state and the virus is currently accountable for millions of infections and hundreds of thousands of demises.

The majority of infected individuals (about 80%) suffer from mild clinical symptoms [2]. Nevertheless, a small percentage may suffer from severe clinical manifestations, especially if they are over 65 years of age or have co-morbidities such as diabetes or hypertension [3]. These individuals frequently have a need for hospitalization and one in five needs intensive care unit (ICU) care [4]. Mortality can be as high as 26.6% in older individuals [5].

As efficacious management for the virus is not yet known, one of the main actions adopted by governments to stop its spread is home confinement of the population and mass restriction of movement. With more than 200 countries in the world affected by the pandemic, these actions have led to major changes in society as a whole. One of the principal repercussions has been a huge increase in the use of digital systems.

The pandemic has exacerbated the crisis of confidence that was already taking place in many health organizations and government institutions. Moreover, another global disaster, in this case the financial crisis that happened in 2008, also drastically diminished people's confidence in governments and institutions for their role in taking care of the crisis. This was one of the chief motives that led Satoshi Nakamoto to publish the article in which he proposed a novel system for establishing mechanisms of confidence in financial markets without the need for the participation of intermediaries such as governments or banks. This system utilized a foundational technology that used distributed ledger of peer-to-peer networks and was called blockchain technology (BCT) [7].

Blockchain Technology (BCT) and COVID-19

BCT and the other cryptocurrencies brought about a radical change in the area of economics. However, the use of BCT surpasses the exclusively economic. Its characteristics make it ideal to be utilized as a decentralized and safe information support system.

BCT can be considered as a distributed database. In each block the updated set of information is saved as well as the whole chronological succession of changes and data on network activity. Blockchain is an increasing list of records called blocks that are connected to each other by cryptographic techniques. Each block includes a cryptographic hash of the prior block, a timestamp and the transaction data. Blockchain systems rely on mining techniques to sum transactions and form the blocks that will be connected to the data stream. Once the transaction is identified by a sufficient number of nodes, it reaches consensus, and turns into a perpetual part of the database [8].

The global pandemic calamity has activated interest in novel technologies and has focused on the many health and economic applications that BCT can have [9]. Nonetheless, as with healthcare, the successful deployment of BCT has need of teamwork in an interdisciplinary approach. Only in this manner can it genuinely help to resolve problems.

BCT can ameliorate global health practice by promoting entry to financing mechanisms, smart contracts, assisting to guard patient privacy, smoothing the referral circuit between health centers and contributing novel payment and reimbursement methods for professionals [10]. This is why BCT could play an important role in countries with fewer health resources.

It is clear that the pandemic has caused alterations in many aspects of daily life that have accentuated new requirements. BCT could help to address many of these novel requirements (Table 5.1). Below are some fields that have been particularly affected by the pandemic and how BCT could help to ameliorate them.

Epidemiological Situation

From an epidemiological point of view, in order to stop the spread of an infectious illness it is essential to rapidly detect the sources of contagion. In the case of Sars-Cov-2, these sources are the infected persons themselves. Besides, it is paramount to determine the contacts these people have had in order to quarantine them and avert outbreaks [11]. Harmonizing detection plans and integrating all this clinical and epidemiological data is a challenge for countries and health organizations. Novel technologies such as BCT can play an important role in ameliorating these aspects [12].

Governments and organizations have used different plans to identify cases and trace their contacts. The chief limiting factor is frequently a country's ability to test [13]. The number of tests carried out is the upper limit that marks the maximum

Table 5.1 Some properties of blockchain technology (BCT) and its possible use in COVID-19 era

Dependable	It avoids the need for third parties as it is completely decentralized. It ameliorates independence from regional or institutional interests
Safe	Encrypted and auditable information without having to access the data itself. Permits the incorporation of sensitive data (including clinical data) while maintaining confidentiality
Differential privacy	It permits the user to be verified without the need for identification. Usefulness in contact tracing
Decentralized	Each user stores the chain. It ameliorates the safety and confidentiality of the information
Immutable	Data can only be modified by the user who has the appropriate key, and the changes are time-stamped. It guarantees the reliability of data, prevents fraud and ameliorates the distribution of chains of goods
Compatible with crypto-currency and smart contracts	It ameliorates the coordination of payments and diminishes costs. Usefulness in new models of labor relations

number of cases that can be identified. In fact, a high percentage of positive testing may denote that not enough cases are being detected [14]. Another paramount element is the neccesity to have the results of the tests available in a short period of time. Ideally, the results should be available within 24 h. There are countries where results take more than 7 days to be attained [14]. In these cases, the transmission chain is so long that it can be intractable.

There are concerns about the ability to identify and report cases, especially with less well resourced health systems with poor laboratory capacity, insufficient surveillance and limited infrastructure as is the case in some African countries. The capacity to precisely diagnose, monitor and report outbreaks necessitates a well resourced and efficacious health system [15]. Many developing countries lack an appropriate epidemiological surveillance system. Besides, they frequently do not have adequate access to health technologies for tracing.

Different countries use distinct plans in the epidemiological control of COVID-19, usually in combination. Most use mobile applications that integrate proximity or geographic location support. Telephone interviewing of patients, families or primary care physicians is also utilized. Some countries, such as South Korea, have analyzed clinical records, closed-circuit video review or credit card transaction history [16]. A complete and strong contact tracing system such as that in South Korea can help control infection, making it easier for other aspects of social life to continue to function. Nevertheless, considerations related to privacy and data processing are the most controversial issues.

The continuous use of mobile phones and Internet-based technologies make it possible to monitor and track people's activities by different actors with not always clear intentions. Due to the pandemic, tracing applications on mobile phones have started to be utilized by many governments to monitor cases. This has caused many organizations and individuals to reveal worries about their confidentiality [17]. This has resulted in a robust interest in technologies that ameliorate the privacy of information such as BCT. It appears clear that the necessity to trace contacts and promote pandemic mitigation actions will endure present for a long time to come.

BCT can ameliorate some aspects of contact tracing by bettering the balance between confidentiality and epidemiological needs. Due to the dual system of public and private keys, BCT permits to collect data from people without compromising their identity [18]. In this manner, people could share their data safely with governments or health institutions without having to identify themselves, ameliorating each individual's control over their own sensitive information.

Another data safety worry is that some applications manage data centrally. Albeit information is frequently saved in anonymized or aggregated form, the likelihood of re-identification is a real peril [19]. BCT, due to its decentralized nature and its differential confidentiality system could ameliorate these aspects.

BCT can also be combined with artificial intelligence to assist health care and epidemiological safety. BCT can ameliorate elements related to electronic clinical records management, drug supply chain management, biomedical investigation, education, distant patient monitoring and health information analysis [20]. It has even been proposed that BCT and artificial intelligence can be integrated within the point of care to permit individuals to test themselves under isolation conditions [21].

As the number of individuals who have been cured of COVID-19 augments, and the likelihood of a vaccine approaches, it may be important to certificate the immune status of each individual. BCT would permit such certification, which could be validated by different government agencies, and would guarantee the confidentiality of other biomedical information [22]. As it is integrated into BCT, this information would be continually refurbished and auditable at all times.

Information Management

In the course of the COVID-19 crisis, a great deal of erroneous or inexact information was generated. In spite of the technical advances available in information technology, there has been tremendous confusion about the true incidence of COVID-19, the number of recorded demises, the efficacy of treatments and the best ways to control the pandemic [22]. The present crisis has demonstrated that effective data sharing is needed to deal with a pandemic. There have also been many defiances related to the appropriate availability of correct information, making it difficult to calculate the number of cases, detect high-risk populations, perform contact tracing operations, and provide required personal protective equipment or

Table 5.2 Characteristics of information during the pandemic and the benefits that blockchain technology (BCT) could bring

Information in COVID-19 ERA	Benefits with BCT
Centralized	Decentralized
Manipulable	Immutable
Heterogeneous	Linked to the chain
Contradictory	Updated
Confusing	Transparent
Dependent on third parties	No trusted intermediaries
Costly	No commissions
No trazability	Auditable

drugs in a coordinated way. All these aspects could have been ameliorated throughout the pandemic if better sources of information had been available [22].

All information on the number of cases and demises that have happened in the course of the pandemic can only be correctly interpreted when clinical context and test results for the virus are integrated. No health organization or country has taken accountability for collecting and reporting data about the pandemic. The available information is scattered across many more or less official websites and documents, displayed in a wide range of configurations.

On the other hand, many institutions acting as trusted parties have promoted the provision of critical services throughout the pandemic. These institutions frequently save information centrally, restraining entry to users and representing a crucial point of information safety failure. Besides, these institutions add expense and time to individual transactions, which can influence efficiency.

BCT can ameliorate data management by individuals, institutions and governments (Table 5.2). It permits to collect data efficiently ensuring the origin of the data, save the information immutably and make an auditable and traceable record over time, registering any modification of the data. This would diminish the peril of data falsification, ameliorating confidence in information providers by promoting non-manipulable, transparent and for all time updated content [23].

Supply Chains

Throughout the COVID-19 pandemic calamity, there have been many difficulties in the supply chains, leading to shortages of some products such as toilet paper and face masks and respirators for hospitals [24]. One of the chief difficulties has been the closure of many factories due to security and epidemiological control issues. Another has been the large discrepancy between the quantities of certain products available and their needs [23].

BCT is ideal to ease the traceability of each good within a supply chain, since each actor involved in that chain uses the same information [25]. The blockchain records are distributed and immutable, being easily auditable at all times. With BCT it is easy to know the state of each good in the supply chain, to estimate the inventory, and to determine an appropriate balance between suppliers and final consumers. Thanks to BCT some tasks that used to take months have been able to be performed in seconds [26]. Its use can make it easier for certain goods to reach the people or organizations that require them most, ameliorating the agility of the distribution chain.

BCT could improve many supply chain issues [27]. In all logistical processes the supply chain frequently works in a standard way. Raw materials are generated, manufactured, stored and then shipped to individual consumers. This would be the flow for normal operation, and would be turned around when returns are made. Besides, all these points in the flow must be subjected to quality control processes.

BCT can be integrated into this process at all points. Each material processed, each equipment utilized or each location where it is operated can generate data that is saved directly in the blockchain. This can be performed in an automated manner without the need for human intervention except in unusual cases [28].

BCT works as a decentralized system in which the different actors implicated in the distribution chain share information while verifying the updated status of this information. Integrated information in the chain would include the available inventory, payments, status of digital assets, logistics and shipping aspects and the recording of transactions. Besides, BCTcan be integrated with other technologies such as cloud computing, sensors or Internet of things to facilitate circuits [29].

It has been described that BCT can promote the adoption of resilient strategies that can ameliorate the cooperation, agility, velocity and visibility of supply chains [30].

During the COVID-19 pandemic, the need to avert counterfeiting and fraud of healthcare products has also appeared [31]. Incorporating BCT into the supply chain would permit real products to be distinguished from counterfeits, as they would be uniquely and unchangeably recognized. This is remarkably useful for goods that have to cross international borders, where heterogeneous checks are performedt. This would ameliorate confidence and diminish fraud and litigation [32]. There are already blockchain-based platforms of this kind in place such as IBM Trust Your Supplier.

Another aspect that has been emphasized during the calamity by COVID-19 has been the potential of initiatives based on circular economy. Circular economy seeks to remove waste and elude wasting materials. It facilitates aspects such as reuse, repair and recycling, through closed circuits that diminish pollution and waste, minimizing the impact on the carbon footprint. Circular economy seeks to preserve the environment while rendering economic benefits [33]. For example, during the pandemic, some distilleries produced disinfectants, and many textile companies' remnants were utilized to make much needed face masks.

This circular economy scenario can also benefit from the utilization of BCT [34]. BCT permits to optimally connect complex multi-level distribution chains, from the most initial phase of production to the final consumer, whilst maintaining circular distribution links [35]. It would therefore be a manner of bringing environmental benefits [36].

Scientific Research

Fraud is not unknown in the history of science. Unfortunately, the calamity related to the pandemic has shown that the repercussions of scientific fraud cannot be accepted.

The amount of scientific papers related to the pandemic has increased a lot in a very short time, with tens of thousands of articles in a few months. A number that is still augmenting. The quality of scientific papers published on this subject is quite different [37].

There is no doubt that researchers have great interest in sharing their work rapidly and openly, in order to get a rapid response and recognition. At the health level this huge amount of papers has happened both in pre-publications and in publications in peer-reviewed scientific journals. In the course of the pandemic at the scientific level one can speak of a true infodemic, a term coined in 2002 by Eysenbach [38].

Due to the tremendous number of papers that have been submitted for review, many journals have had to diminish the time spent on pre-manual assessment. Fourteen medical journals have lessend the time spent on average by 50% on the publication of pandemic articles, thus reducing the time spent on the peer review process [39].

Evidence of these drawbacks, which have been seen in the publication of scientific journals, can be found in a recent case. Two papers were published in prestigious medical journals that had to be withdrawn just a few weeks later. The first paper was published in New England on May 1, 2020, and discussed the lack of adverse effects of ACE inhibitors and angiotensin receptor blockers in individuals with COVID-19 [40]. The second article, published on 22 May 2020 in the Lancet, discussed the potential perils of using chloroquine or hydroxychloroquine for the management of COVID-19 [41]. The two papers shared several of their authors and utilized the same source of information from the data analyzed, an external company called Surgisphere. When other scientists expressed doubts about the nature of the information analyzed, neither the authors nor Surgisphere were able to provide the required evidence to support the outcomes of their work. This confirmed the suspicions that the information had been manipulated and the journals withdrew the papers.

Problems with the validity of published articles are not new, nor have they emerged because of the pandemic. However, these recent events have emphasized the problems in the process of validating and reporting scientific work. Nevertheless, there have already been other cases of publication fraud that have had important consequences. On 28 February 1998 the Lancet published an article connecting vaccination against measles, mumps and rubella to problems of autism and intestinal sickness in 12 children [42]. Subsequent studies encountered no causal relationship, until Wakefield's original paper was withdrawn 12 years later in 2010 [43].

Wakefield's lack of ethics during his research caused tremendous damage, the repercussions of which are still being experienced today. His paper caused vaccination rates to decline and led to mistrust of the work of health organizations. These negative feelings towards vaccines are still observed today, and their repercussions are still being suffered even during the current pandemic.

These problems of fraud or misconduct in the analysis of scientific information are intimately related to the very process of research in today's science. A standard research process is based on data obtained from an individual (usually a patient) who experiences a health intervention. This intervention is measured and analyzed by an intermediary (a researcher) who collects the information to be measured in the study. Another researcher will be accountable for analyzing this data and attaining the outcomes of the intervention. The work performed subsequently is published by the research team and submitted to a journal which must review it. The review process is carried out by peers, i.e. other knowledgeable professionals in the field, who have criteria to detect whether or not the research carried out meets the required quality standards.

When the article is published in a scientific journal, it will be read by professionals and health authorities who will incorporate or not this proposed intervention into daily clinical practice. This would be the manner to close the cycle and the benefits of the research would return to patients themselves.

This process, therefore, needs the involvement of a large number of actors, some of whom are unknown, so it is easy for the information to be modified during the process of attaining it or during the subsequent analysis process [44]. When this process fails repeatedly, mistrust of the process itself is produced.

To diminish the number of mistakes journals may require submission of original information for parallel analysis, in-depth revision of the study protocol and statistical analysis, or a thorough research of potential conflicts of interest of the authors. Nonetheless, none of this guarantees that fraud in the publication of scientific papers will not happen again. This problem is aggravated during a pandemic such as COVID-19, where much remains to be understood [37].

BCT could ameliorate the whole data processing processrequired in scientific research. BCT generates a distributed ledger that guarantees the immutability, transparency and traceability of the information even between two or more distant parties with no mutual confidence [45].

Currently, the databases utilized in research are contained in devices or in individual cloud. The various researchers enter the outcomes of their research into this database in parallel. A major advantage of BCT would be that the entire research database would be saved on each of the researchers' devices. Moreover, all data entered (anonymized at source) would be automatically synchronized and all these operations would be traceable and safe due to the blockchain characteristics [37].

Within BCT, public (permissionless ledger) and private (permissioned ledger) variants have been utilized. The best known public option would be bitcoin. This is an open solution that does not need authorization by a third party and is not controlled by a single entity. One problem with the public ledger is that transactions are visible to everyone, so privacy could be jeopardized. Additionally, this type of chain is based on consensus algorithms, so its utilization may be difficult when the number of users is very low, as is commonly the case when a scientific paper is published [46].

On the other hand, private chains are based on closed networks. These systems benefit from the distributed nature of blockchain, sharing the ledger with all users of the network, but with the benefits of a completely traceable and immutable database. Private blockchain depends on a mechanism called selective endorsement, in which some predetermined endorsers are accountable for corroborating or invalidating a transaction. For this reason, this type of private solution permits transactions to be made in less time and with less computing power than public ones [47]. Due to these characteristics, a private solution is presumably better suited to be utilized in the scientific research process. In fact, some initiatives of this kind are already being adopted [48].

Therefore BCTcould have an important place in corroborating the whole process of scientific research. It would be a manner of ensuring the integrity of the information, while addressing the complex ethical challenges implicated in research

The Working Model

Mitigation actions taken during the pandemic such as lockdown or social distancing have augmented the utilization of internet services from 40 to 100% compared to pre-pandemic levels. The efficiency of many workers depends on their capacity to connect to the Internet, and during the pandemic this aspect has only augmented. Some video conferencing services such as Zoom have risen their use tenfold [49].

During the pandemic, some countries have restrained access to the Internet [50]. Regulation of Internet access and bandwidth usage has been a key issue during the Covid calamity, and forthcoming regulation by individual governments will be crucial. Those without an Internet connection risk exclusion from employment [51].

The way many professionals work has changed entirely. Novel recommendations for novel working models have appeared, changing from the office to the home and from face-to-face to virtual meetings. This new model of home-based teleworking is being chosen by many corporations. On the other hand, some enterprises are employing workers for specific tasks, with very short contracts, in an informal manner. Well-known examples are Uber and Glovo. This novel nature of the working relationship generates novel necessities for workers, both from a psychological point of view and in terms of technical support and design of their own working model. Aspects related to new working models must be addressed in an adequate manner [6].

One of the fields of work that has experienced the most radical change during the pandemic has been education. Many schools, universities and training associations have been obliged to make an epitome shift from a face-to-face training model to a tele-training model. Many of these associations have changed to video conferencing platforms or to asynchronous training models [52].

This new model of distance working from home has been associated with ameliorated efficiency, but also with an augmentation in techno-stress. Furthermore, the constant use of video-conferencing tools makes the worker feel under endless surveillance, and all interactions are "hyper-focused" [53]. The new worker who carries out his or her function from home have to learn new technologies, stay connected at all times, be available for work on a constant basis and deal multitasking.

Many of the problems related to the homework model include aspects of confidence, efficacious communication, performance measurement and cooperation. All these aspects can be ameliorated with the use of BCT.

BCT can also provide access to smart contracts [54]. Smart Contracts are computerized protocols that promote, authenticate, or reinforce the negotiation of an accord. These accords permit agreements to be reached between different users of the network, without the implication of trusted third parties. These accords are transparent and can be refined and sequenced in detail. In today's fast-changing labor market environment, smart contracts could provide safety for workers and enterprises while maintaining the required operational flexibility.

In spite of the numerous possibilities of BCT in the working environment, in order to be adjusted effectively, it must be integrated into the different workflows of workers and enterprises. Nonetheless, because of its many advantages it could be utilized still in resource-scarce environments such as developing countries [23].

Finances

BCT was originally created as a monetary system, so it is not surprising that it was utilized for this aim during the pandemic. BCT can ameliorate entry to financing systems by permitting multilateral mechanisms, constructing new markets, adopting Smart contracts and creating novel forms of payment to professionals. This could have a tremendous impact on patients, institutions and countries themselves [55].

Novel technologies can ameliorate payments between users in different countries, providing faster, cheaper and safer ways of payment than those currently available. Blockchain's capacity to operate in a decentralized way diminishes dependence on trusted third parties, saving costs by decreasing fees to almost 0% [56].

The likelihood of BCT to include smart contracts can permit organizations to ameliorate financing circuits. For example, it is feasible to guarantee the services performed, the costs incurred, even the result attained, and connect this entire data set to a specific payment. Because of the immutable and time-stamped nature of the transactions performed through BCT, it could help to diminish mistakes and reduce fraud [57].

During the pandemic, two circumstances have appeared that are directly related to monetary aspects. On the one hand, the use of money in banknotes and coins has been restrained because of the likelihood that they could act as a fomite and become objects of contagion. On the other hand, because of the many labor problems enforced by confinement during the pandemic, many governments have provided funds and assistance to mitigate the socio-economic consequences. Many of these funds and support have been provided through digital transfers and payment applications.

Financial aid and the whole donation process (storage, logistics and distribution) can be done through BCT. It is a manner to ameliorate their efficiency, diminsh fraud and strengthen social cohesion. In fact, during the pandemic, blockchain-based platforms such as hyperchain have been utilized for this purpose [58].

Conclusions

The coronavirus pandemic has caused a major calamity, and like any calamity, has produced a number of needs. New technologies can be utilized to meet these needs and mitigate some of the problems related to the pandemic. BCT permits to store data in an immutable manner establishing a temporary record of any modification made. Besides, it works in a decentralized, safe, independent of trusted third parties and maintaining the confidentiality of the information stored in it. All these characteristics have led to an increasing interest in many social and health areas and to the existence of more and more platforms that successfully use it. Some of its applications with great potential for development would be epidemiological monitoring, supply chains, information management, scientific research, new work or financial models.

References

1. Lipsitch M, Swerdlow DL, Finelli L (2020) Defining the epidemiology of Covid-19-Studies needed. N Engl J Med 382:1194–1196
2. Rodriguez-Morales AJ, Cardona-Ospina JA, Gutiérrez-Ocampo E, Villamizar-Peña R, Holguin-Rivera Y, Escalera-Antezana JP et al (2020) Latin American network of coronavirus disease 2019-COVID-19 research (LANCOVID-19). Electronic address: https://www.lancovid.org. Clinical, laboratory and imaging features of COVID-19: a systematic review and meta-analysis. Travel Med Infect Dis 34:101623
3. CDC COVID-19 Response Team (2020) Severe outcomes among patients with coronavirus disease 2019 (COVID-19)-United States, February 12–March 16, 2020. MMWR Morb Mortal Wkly Rep 69:343–6
4. Simpson R, Robinson L (2020) Rehabilitation after critical illness in people with COVID-19 infection. Am J Phys Med Rehabil 99:470–474
5. Kang SJ, Jung SI (2020) Age-related morbidity and mortality among patients with COVID-19. Infect Chemother 52:154–164

6. De' R, Pandey N, Pal A (2020) Impact of digital surge during Covid-19 pandemic: a viewpoint on research and practice. Int J Inf Manage 55:102171
7. Bohannon J (2016) The bitcoin busts. Science 351(6278):1144–1146
8. Crosby M, Pattanayak P, Verma S, Kalyanaraman V (2016) Section technology: beyond bitcoin. Appl Innov Rev 2:6–10
9. Wladawsky-Berger I (May 01, 2020) Blockchain may offer solutions to fighting Covid-19. Wall Street J. https://www.wsj.com/articles/blockchain-may-offer-solutions-to-fighting-covid-19-01588351297. Accessed 11.11.20
10. Resiere D, Resiere D, Kallel H (2020) Implementation of medical and scientific cooperation in the Caribbean using blockchain technology in Coronavirus (Covid-19) pandemics. J Med Syst 44:123
11. Dhama K, Khan S, Tiwari R, Sircar S, Bhat S, Malik YS et al (2020) Coronavirus disease 2019-COVID-19. Clin Microbiol Rev 33:e00028-e120
12. Roman-Belmonte JM, De la Corte-Rodriguez H, Rodriguez-Merchan EC (2018) How blockchain technology can change medicine. Postgrad Med 130:420–427
13. Salathé M, Althaus CL, Neher R, Stringhini S, Hodcroft E, Fellay J et al (2020) COVID-19 epidemic in Switzerland: on the importance of testing, contact tracing and isolation. Swiss Med Wkly 150:w20225
14. Hasell J, Mathieu E, Beltekian D, Macdonald B, Giattino C, Ortiz-Ospina E et al (2020) A cross-country database of COVID-19 testing. Sci Data. 7:345
15. Rattanaumpawan P, Boonyasiri A, Vong S, Thamlikitkul V (2018) Systematic review of electronic surveillance of infectious diseases with emphasis on antimicrobial resistance surveillance in resource-limited settings. Am J Infect Control 46:139–146
16. COVID-19 National Emergency Response Center, Epidemiology and Case Management Team, Korea Centers for Disease Control and Prevention. Coronavirus Disease-19: the first 7,755 cases in the Republic of Korea. Osong Public Health Res Perspect (2020 Apr) 11 (2):85–90
17. Bradford L, Aboy M, Liddell K (2020) COVID-19 contact tracing apps: a stress test for privacy, the GDPR, and data protection regimes. J Law Biosci 7:lsaa034
18. Xu L, Shah N, Chen L, Diallo N, Gao S, Lu Y et al (2017) Enabling the sharing economy: privacy respecting contract based on public blockchain. In: BCC '17: proceedings of the ACM workshop on blockchain, cryptocurrencies and contracts. 2017 presented at: BCC 2017: ACM workshop on blockchain, cryptocurrencies and contracts, April 2, 2017, Abu Dhabi, pp 15–21
19. Arriagada-Bruneau G, Müller VC, Gilthorpe MS (2020) The ethical imperatives of the COVID 19 pandemic: a review from data ethics. Veritas: Revista de Filosofía y Teología 46:13–35
20. Agbo CC, Mahmoud QH, Eklund JM (2019) Blockchain technology in healthcare: a systematic review. Healthcare (Basel) 7:56
21. Mashamba-Thompson TP, Crayton ED (2020) Blockchain and artificial intelligence technology for novel coronavirus sisease-19 self-testing. Diagnostics (Basel) 10:198
22. Khurshid A (2020) Applying blockchain technology to address the crisis of trust during the COVID-19 pandemic. JMIR Med Inform 8:e20477
23. Marbouh D, Abbasi T, Maasmi F, Omar IA, Debe MS, Salah K et al (2020) Blockchain for COVID-19: review, opportunities, and a trusted tracking system. Arab J Sci Eng 12:1–17
24. Lancet T (2020) Editorial: COVID-19: protecting health-care workers. Lancet 395 (10228):922
25. Min H (2019) Blockchain technology for enhancing supply chain resilience. Bus Horiz 62:35–45
26. Yiannas F (2018) A new era of food transparency powered by blockchain. Innov Technol Gov Glob 12:46–56

27. Kuupiel D, Bawontuo V, Mashamba-Thompson TP (2017) Improving the accessibility and efficiency of point-of-care diagnostics services in low- and middle-income countries: lean and agile supply chain management. Diagnostics (Basel) 7:58
28. Kho JS, Jeong J (2020) HACCP-based cooperative model for smart factory in South Korea. Procedia Comput Sci 175:778–783
29. Treiblmaier H, Mirkovski K, Lowry PB, Zacharia ZG (2020) The physical internet as a new supply chain paradigm: a systematic literature review and a comprehensive framework. Int J Logist Manage 31:239–287
30. Kalla A, Hewa T, Mishra RA, Ylianttila M, Liyanage M (2020) The role of blockchain to fight against COVID-19. IEEE Eng Manage Rev 48:85–96
31. OECD/EUIPO (2020) Trade in counterfeit pharmaceutical products, illicit trade. OECD Publishing, Paris. https://doi.org/10.1787/a7c7e054-en
32. Kumar R, Tripathi R (2019) Traceability of counterfeit medicine supply chain through Blockchain. In: 2019 presented at: 11th international conference on communication systems & networks (COMSNETS), January 7–11, 2019, Bengaluru, India
33. Morseletto P (2020) Targets for a circular economy. Resour Conserv Recycl 153:104553
34. Nandi S, Sarkis J, Hervani AA, Helms MM (2021) Redesigning supply chains using blockchain-enabled circular economy and COVID-19 experiences. Sustain Prod Consum 27:10–22
35. Saberi S, Kouhizadeh M, Sarkis J, Shen L (2019) Blockchain technology and its relationships to sustainable supply chain management. Int J Prod Res 57:2117–2135
36. Kouhizadeh M, Saberi S, Sarkis J (2021) Blockchain technology and the sustainable supply chain: theoretically exploring adoption barriers. Int J Prod Econ 231:107831
37. Boetto E, Golinelli D, Carullo G, Fantini MP (2020) Frauds in scientific research and how to possibly overcome them. J Med Ethics 1–5
38. Eysenbach G (2020) How to fight an infodemic: the four pillars of infodemic management. J Med Internet Res 22:e21820
39. Horbach SPJM (2020) Pandemic publishing: medical journals drastically speed up their publication process for Covid-19. bioRxiv 2020.04.18.045963. https://doi.org/10.1101/2020.04.18.045963
40. Mehra MR, Desai SS, Kuy S, Henry TD, Patel AN (2020) Retraction-Cardiovascular disease, drug therapy, and mortality in Covid-19. N Engl J Med 382:2582
41. Mehra MR, Desai SS, Ruschitzka F, Patel AN (1820) Retraction-Hydroxychloroquine or chloroquine with or without a macrolide for treatment of COVID-19: a multinational registry analysis. Lancet 2020:395
42. Wakefield AJ, Murch SH, Anthony A, Linnell J, Casson DM, Malik M et al (1998) Retracted-Ileal-lymphoid-nodular hyperplasia, non-specific colitis, and pervasive developmental disorder in children. Lancet 351:637–641
43. Godlee F, Smith J, Marcovitch H (2011) Wakefield's article linking MMR vaccine and autism was fraudulent. BMJ 342:c7452
44. Moore N, Juillet Y, Bertoye PH; Round Table No 4, Giens XXII (2007) Integrity of scientific data: transparency of clinical trial data. Therapie 62:203–9, 211–6
45. Mackey TK, Shah N, Miyachi K et al (2019) A framework proposal for Blockchain-Based scientific publishing using shared governance. Frontiers in Blockchain 2:19
46. Choudhury O, Fairoza N, Sylla I, Das A (2020) A Blockchain framework for managing and monitoring data in multi-site clinical trials 1–13. https://arxiv.org/pdf/1902.03975.pdf
47. Pandey P, Litoriya R (2020) Promoting trustless computation through blockchain technology [published online ahead of print, 2020 May 20]. Natl Acad Sci Lett 1–7
48. Wong DR, Bhattacharya S, Butte AJ (2019) Prototype of running clinical trials in an untrustworthy environment using blockchain. Nat Commun 10:917
49. Branscombe M (2020) The network impact of the global COVID-19 pandemic. April 14, Accessed June 6, 2020, from The New Stack. https://thenewstack.io/the-networkimpact-of-the-global-covid-19-pandemic/

50. Chhibber M (2020) Militancy in Kashmir peaked without 4G, but Modi govt keeps forgetting this in court. May 6, Accessed June 6, 2020, from The Print. https://theprint.in/opinion/militancy-in-kashmir-peaked-without-4g-but-modi-govt-keeps-forgettingthis-in-court/415072/
51. Ahmed W, Vidal-Alaball J, Downing J, López SF (2020) COVID-19 and the 5G conspiracy theory: social network analysis of twitter data. J Med Internet Res 22:e19458
52. Muflih S, Abuhammad S, Karasneh R, Al-Azzam S, Alzoubi KH, Muflih M (2020) Online education for undergraduate health professional education during the COVID-19 pandemic: attitudes, barriers, and ethical issues. Res Sq [Preprint]. Jul 16:rs.3.rs-42336. https://doi.org/10.21203/rs.3.rs-42336/v1
53. Bondanini G, Giorgi G, Ariza-Montes A, Vega-Muñoz A, Andreucci-Annunziata P (2020) Technostress dark side of technology in the workplace: a scientometric analysis. Int J Environ Res Public Health 17:8013
54. Szabo N (1997) Formalizing and securing relationships on public networks. First Monday 2 (9). https://doi.org/10.5210/fm.v2i9.548
55. Till BM, Peters AW, Afshar S, Meara JG, Meara J (2017) From blockchain technology to global health equity: can cryptocurrencies finance universal health coverage? Published correction appears in BMJ Glob Health 2:e000570
56. Pisa M, Juden M (2017) Blockchain and economic development: Hype vs. Reality. Center for global development policy paper, 107. https://www.cgdev.org/sites/default/files/blockchain-and-economic-development-hype-vs-reality_0.pdf
57. The Financial Cost of Healthcare Fraud (2011) What data from around the world shows. University of Portsmouth, Centre for count fraud studies, 1–20. https://www.quotidianosanita.it/allegati/allegato6444539.pdf
58. Chang V, Baudier P, Zhang H, Xu Q, Zhang J, Arami M (2020) How Blockchain can impact financial services-the overview, challenges and recommendations from expert interviewees. Technol Forecast Soc Change 158:120166

Distributed Ledgers and Immunity Passports: The Intersection of Clinical Medicine and Digital Technology

6

Michael S. Firstenberg, Benjamin A. Wilson, Dianne E. McCallister, and Stanislaw P. Stawicki

> *In any bureaucracy, there's a natural tendency to let the system become an excuse for inaction.*
>
> –Chris Fussell

Abstract

As the world continues to adapter to the complex challenges that have evolved as a consequence of the COVID-19 pandemic—and the efforts used to minimize viral spread, the idea of an immunity passport has evolved to allow for those to can demonstrate they present minimal risk of transmission (or acquiring) of disease while allowing for resumption of social interactions and activities. Coronavirus immunity passports, much like conventional visas and passports, and existing vaccination records that are often required for social interactions (travel, attending school, healthcare employment, etc.), are currently being developed. However, as we hope to address in this chapter, there are extensive challenges to successful global implementation. In addition to socio-economic challenges, there are substantial concerns of individual privacy, integrity and accuracy of the data especially in the context of known biology of infection, viral

M. S. Firstenberg (✉)
William Novick Global Cardiac Alliance, Memphis, TN, USA
e-mail: msfirst@gmail.com

B. A. Wilson
Blockchain-as-a-Service Company, San Francisco, CA, USA

D. E. McCallister
Diagnosis Well, Inc., Greenwood Village, CO, USA

S. P. Stawicki
Department of Research & Innovation, St. Luke's University Health Network, Bethlehem, PA 18015, USA

mutation, and human immune system function, costs, and overall practical feasibility. The use of blockchain technologies, as we discuss, might help address some of these challenges and allow for successful widespread acceptance and use. Systemic and processes that combine the technologies and benefits of a blockchain with the scientific principles vaccination and immune biology might reflect the ideal approach to this global problem.

Keywords

Blockchain · Immunity passports · COVID-19 · Immunology · Vaccination · Privacy · Coronavirus

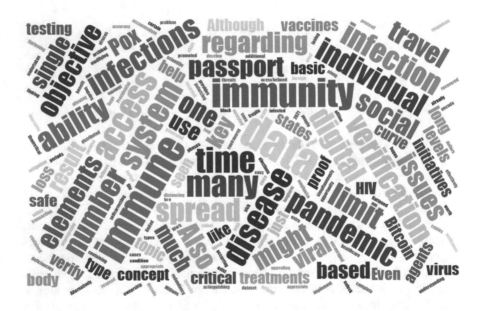

Introduction

In December 2020, the United Kingdom and the United States almost simultaneously provided a governmental stamp of approval (as emergency use authorizations) for the first vaccines against severe acute respiratory syndrome coronavirus 2 (SARS-CoV-2), the novel coronavirus associated with coronavirus disease 2019 (COVID-19) infections. Around the world, regulatory and governmental approvals were quickly implemented to provide all available vaccines in a highly prioritized fashion. It is important to remember that these approvals occurred just over a year after the first reported case in the current pandemic (circa December 2019) and was set amidst rapidly escalating infections—and deaths—worldwide in both high-income and low-and-middle-income countries. While the facts regarding the etiology, transmission, political, socio-economic, and scientific details of this unquestionable global health disaster will be debated for decades to come, what is clear is the vast spectrum of implications impacting all walks of human life— particularly in regards to how we approach and interact with each other.

During the course of the pandemic numerous initiatives were implemented at various levels of society by politicians, industry leaders, and healthcare experts in efforts to control the spread of the virus and to limit infections and their associated complications [1]. The initial goal was referred to as "flattening the curve"—a concept in global health in which the focus is to minimize the initial simultaneous huge number of acute cases which would overwhelm a healthcare system and the ability to appropriately care for the ill [2]. It was accepted that although the actual number of "sick or infected" people might be the same with a "flattened curve," the number of cases would be distributed over time, allowing for an already fragile healthcare system to effectively accommodate more patients over a period of time, rather than being overwhelmed by huge influxes over short periods of time. The other theoretical benefit of the "flattening the curve" approach is that it provides the scientific and medical community with the opportunity and extra time to develop appropriate treatments and implement key mitigation measures. Work can then proceed on potential curative treatments, disease modifying agents or vaccines, all in the hopes of containing and then extinguishing the pandemic. Although appealing in concept, the initiatives undertaken are not without important conse- quences at all levels.

The focus of the current chapter is not to debate these initiatives, which are associated with some degree of controversy (despite being implemented to control the spread of the virus) but rather to highlight the fact that disease containment was a key principle in this context. These initiatives, focused on reducing or stopping viral transmission, emphasized the role of social distancing as a means of trying to prevent the spread of COVID-19 infections, from person-to-person-to-community-to-soci- ety, as much as possible. Again, while many of the specific actions varied across the world, and many generated intense social debate, scrutiny, and even riots and rebellion; the reality quickly became a fundamental shift in the social contract as it applies to all aspects of human interactions.

The extent and magnitude of the social distancing initiatives, which included such measures as closing restaurants, bars, and clubs, working remotely from home, minimizing travel (especially non-local/interstate), closing in-person schools and educational offerings, foregoing business meetings and in-person sporting and cultural events, and a transitioning from these interactions to a digital domain with online meetings and virtual encounters becoming wide-spread. While the effects (both successes and failures) of these major shifts in activities were appealing to some and devastating to others, their effectiveness was highly questioned as many areas of the world experienced multiple waves and recurrent spikes of infections and increasing number of cases. Nevertheless, such initiatives quickly became the "new normal" with regards to how humanity transitioned to different "functional levels" across the world with the primary goal of minimization, at all levels of society, the spread of the virus from those who are infected to those who are not. [Note: It is important to emphasize that social distancing, again a topic that generated much controversy—especially since much of the acute phases of the pandemic in the United States were occurring simultaneously along one of the most polarizing Presidential elections—was only one of many initiatives promoted and encouraged to limit viral transmission].

Whether effective or ineffective, at some point, society must evolve toward a state in which human-human interactions can and should occur at a certain generally expected, minimal level. Regardless of the economic implications, humans are social creatures and to be emotionally healthy, we must be able to travel, go to school, attend events, go to work and be productive, and do so by interacting in person in addition to the virtual or digital online domain [3]. This raises the fundamental question of how can we return to in-person interactions in a safe manner that limits the spread of infections, such as COVID-19 and also allows people to feel adequate controls are in place to help them feel psychologically safe with these in-person interactions despite perceptions of actual and theoretical risks.

The concept of developing a mechanism by which it can easily be determined who is "safe" or "not safe" to interact within a society (travel, work, school, sporting events, etc.) is not novel. Passports of "various sorts" have been developed and are in routine use across different domains of our lives. Such passports allow for safe and expedient vetting of those who are deemed to be safe to enter a different country or any designated area within a specific region. Regardless of whether it is traveling internationally or proving your age to enter a bar or a concert, these systems already exist, are widely accepted by the population as specific implementations of a system that facilitates that attainment of certain goals or objectives.

Vaccines and Immunity

While it is important to recognize that vaccines and immunity are not always synonymous. The presence of a vaccination does not guarantee immunity, nor does immunity negate the need for vaccination. It is also important to recognize that vaccinations are an essential part of our overall public health and safety system, and there are numerous examples of this. For example, children cannot go to school, in many countries around the world, without proof of vaccination or immunity to many common childhood infections—such as chicken pox, diphtheria, pertussis, tetanus, measles, mumps, and rubella. Healthcare workers are required to demonstrate vaccination (and often immunity) to influenza and hepatitis B.

On a global scale, many areas of the world require documentation of vaccination to Yellow Fever and evidence to document the level of risk for transmitting tuberculosis, as dictated by local governmental entities prior to entry into the country. Moreover, these specific rules and requirements may vary from country to country and even between specific regions within a country. While the science in which these policies are based and the methods used to verify the source data documenting immunity, exposure, previous infection, or vaccination, are open to much interpretation and debate, they do exist and are strictly enforced. Hence, the growing concern that a requirement for "proof of immunity" before engaging in a social activity or participating openly in society raises the need that this proof is appropriately documented and that a chain of custody is present that verifies the accuracy, integrity, and appropriateness of the data. Moreover, this needs to be implemented in a reproducible fashion across different societies, cultures, and governmental entities.

Equally important is the issue regarding protecting the privacy of the data, at the individual and societal level as well as the protection of the "owners" of the data and the processes used to collect, maintain, and share such data be protected, against inappropriate uses [4]. Regardless of how this is defined, there will also be legitimate privacy concerns that those in power, or seeking economic or political power, might use such data to their socio-economic, political, cultural, religious, advantage. Hence a question arises, how can such data be protected in a manner in which it is only used for a common good? Examples of this concept include the laws in the United States that were enacted as part of the Health Insurance Portability and Accountability Act of 1996 (HIPAA) and that define the limits and penalties regarding access to healthcare information and limit use [5, 6]. While such laws have been enforced and found to be useful, at least in the United States, there are no such global protections in place and even in the US, there are concerns about how to balance the protection of an individual's privacy with regards to health risks to the needs of society to use such data for a common good.

COVID-19 contact tracing and exposure notifications are just one of many concepts that have evolved in the debate regarding an individual's privacy and concerns about personal data being used to discriminate versus the social needs to use such data to limit the spread of a deadly infection [1, 7]. Regardless of the ethics, morality, and politics of such tracking activities—all critically important concepts that are beyond the scope of this chapter, it is important that proper tools be developed and used to help not only solve the fundamental problems, but also address some of the obvious concerns. Morality aside (at least for the time being)—even though no tool or process will be perfect—it is important to recognize many of the complex issues that must be at least acknowledged before wide-spread, if not global, adoption.

Basics of Blockchain Theory and Technologies

The concept of a blockchain—not to be confused with cryptocurrencies (i.e., Bitcoin) that utilize blockchain technology and related techniques—represents an innovative tool for maintaining data integrity, privacy, access, and scale that might be uniquely suited for use with immunity passports [8, 9]. For the sake of clarity, all cryptocurrencies have a blockchain, but not all blockchains are associated with a cryptocurrency. The focus of the current discussion is the blockchain technology. At its core, a blockchain is an immutable ledger of data which when applied to cryptocurrencies, provides a reliable and reproducible history of financial transactions over time that clearly documents ownership [10]. More generally, by design and implementation, a blockchain ledger provides fundamental mechanisms that ensure privacy, accuracy and integrity of data, and ease of access. While the technical aspects of how a blockchain works are extremely complex, the concept is an extension of the evolving concepts of maintaining data integrity and protecting against malicious use or corruption of such data.

In general, and in brief, a data element (like a record of a financial transaction between 2 people) is stored in a transaction within a given block [9]. A block is a page of a ledger book, a "database" being able to store many thousands, if not millions, of data elements (called transactions in the blockchain vernacular). Each transaction is encoded in such a way that the dataset can be easily verified. This allows for rapid verification against fraud and errors. In order to execute a transaction, "Unspent Outputs" (known under the acronym "UTXO") are sent to other addresses after authentication by the original owner. Without revealing passcodes, others can verify that the transaction was completed in a protocol-compliant manner. Such "Unspent Outputs" are protected and encrypted by a private key/ public key combination—similar to how in a bank, there is public access to the bank, and there is only private access to account information or to a safety deposit box. With access to both the private and public keys, transactions can be issued, data can be stored and ownership can be confirmed or verified [11]. The public and private keys are long alphanumeric strings that have built in verification checks. If a holder of UTXO authorizes a transaction, the private key is all that is necessary. If possession of the private key is ever lost, control of the UTXO is also lost [12].

Hence, an individual's proof of ownership of data (for example, a certain amount of cryptocurrency) is linked to the ability to supply a private and public key to 'unlock' the UTXO that resides in a particular block on that particular blockchain [13]. While the number of private key permutations is finite, the number of combinations is sufficiently large to virtually never pose a risk of a "collision" in reuse. The public and private keys are generated with an algorithm that allows the value to check for validity, meaning the strings have encoding requirements much like the Luhn Formula [14, 15] used to create credit card numbers. The permutations of keys are essentially endless and much like credit card and social security (at least as used in the United States) numbers have systems encoded into them to ensure accuracy and limited tampering and fraud. Analogous mechanisms are designed into the private keys to help validate the integrity of the blockchain key. Similarly, each block is then hashed with a computational algorithm to yield a lengthy alphanumeric code. This is called a Merkle Tree [16, 17] and results in a Merkle Root value that represents each distinct block (or page of the ledger book). Even the slightest change, such as a single digit, in a block, when hashed will result in a completely different Merkle Root [18]. If, when hashed, a code from a block of data does not match the hash code as stored in a different block (i.e., the block created immediately after a proceeding block is complete), it is implied that the block is no longer accurate and has been potentially, maliciously or accidentally, corrupted. Redundancies of blocks across the network then allow for self-correction of corrupted blocks to maintain, automatically and inherently, data accuracy across the entire virtual construct.

As the overall chain of blocks grows (e.g., hence the term 'blockchain') the data stored in individual blocks serves to verify and preserve the accuracy of the encrypted data elements contained in the preceding block. Furthermore, again by design, copies of the entire blockchain can—and are—stored in virtual locations throughout the world (and hence the term 'distributed ledger') [19, 20]. Copies of a blockchain, as recorded at any moment in time, can also be saved as a digital file, off-line, for additional redundancy and long-term archival of critical data. As long as two or more copies of the blockchain exist, a self-correcting mechanism can help verify the accuracy of the data and as long as the cryptography can be used to encode and decode with both public and private keys to unlock the data, individual data elements can be recovered. Alternatively, losing one's private key—the only tool linking to a specific record of a transaction or dataset contained within a block —will result in complete loss of access to that data and, thereby, proof of ownership. Millions of dollars' worth of Bitcoin and other cryptocurrencies have been lost when private keys have been lost or inadvertently destroyed [12]. Since the entire system is so secure, once a private key is lost, access or proof of ownership is also gone—forever.

While the technologies and tools of blockchain may be sophisticated, especially with regards to the creation of the blocks and the links to cryptocurrencies, the fundamental principles as applied to data ownership, redundancy, accuracy, and integrity are sound and currently serve as the foundation for a substantial (over USD 2 trillion in market capitalization as of April 2021 and rising quickly) growing financial set of tools both for investment and commerce.

In addition to an understanding of how blockchain technologies might be applied to tracking one's immune status, it is also important to understand the basic principles of how the human immune system works with regards to identifying "foreign" (i.e., infectious agents) from "self". The ability to separate "self" from "non-self" and mount a corresponding response to limit the disease and any associated infectious complications and transmission, while allowing for "exposure recall," are the primary functions of the human immune-response system [21–23]. It is this "memory of exposure" that serves as the basis for the concept of immunity by attenuating the consequences of either a primary, first-time, exposure or subsequent re-infections. The understanding of the complexities of this cellular and protein-mediated system, including feedback loops, redundancies, and modifiable degrees of response over time has resulted in numerous Nobel Prizes and advances in medicine that have enabled revolutionary therapies ranging from vaccinations allowing disease eradication to the ability to perform organ transplantation. The significance and intricacies of the human immune system cannot be overstated nor adequately explained in the context of a single chapter, but an understanding of fundamental principles should be required of all students of the biological sciences.

Basics of the Human Immune System

While the human immune system is extremely complex—and a thorough review is beyond the scope of this chapter—the basic principles of its function are based upon a foreign substance, considered "an antigen," being recognized by the immune system as "foreign" which then elicits a cellular response by producing specific proteins, called "antibodies" [24]. These generally highly specific "antibodies" then target and bind to the "antigens" to form an "antigen-antibody complex" [25]. These complexes then activate various cellular components of the immune system via a very complex process which then serves to eliminate from the body these "foreign" complexes. This highly biologically regulated system, using various feedback mechanisms, also has a "memory" component to its functionality —specifically, the initial response to a foreign agent (antigen) is different from the immune system response if the organism is re-exposed or re-challenged again at a later time [21, 24].

In the context of bacterial or viral infection, typically the "antigen" is a specific protein complex on the cell surface (for bacteria) or part of the capsule (for viruses) that is recognized as being "foreign." Much like how many automobiles are recognized specifically by their hood ornaments, foreign objects are similarly recognized by only a small identifying protein structure—"antigens." Rarely do different biological objects share similar "antigens," but such occurrences do sxist in nature. Unfortunately, infectious agents—again, such as bacteria and viruses, can evolve or mutate in manners in which their antigens change or mutate over time. These changes in "antigens" over time, often considered an extension of Darwin's "survival of the fittest" theories, can result in a reinfection from a previously exposed virus, resulting in an "immune response" similar to the initial exposure. This adaptive mechanism of bacteria and viruses helps to explain why certain diseases, such as varicella zoster (the viral that causes Chicken Pox) rarely cause a second infection while viruses that cause the "seasonal flu" or the "common cold" are constantly mutating the antigen protein structures in a manner that can result in repeated re-infections [26–28].

While this system is highly effective, the initial response and the re-exposure response to various "foreign agents" can be highly variable and unpredictable. Occasionally, the body's response can be more detrimental than the impact of the foreign infection itself. For example, while no doubt painful, a first bee sting, in some people, can be relatively minor, while the consequences of a second or third sting can be a life-threatening event [29]. This concept serves as the basis for allergic reactions—a response to previous exposures can range from minor symptoms such as redness, swelling, discomfort, low-grade fevers and chills to major consequences such as severe cardiovascular collapse and even mortality.

In addition, as efficient as the immune system usually functions, there are a variety of well-known disease states that illustrate some of the problems and consequences that can occur when this highly-evolved system does not work properly. For example, there are a variety of auto-immune disorders in which the immune system recognizes intrinsic cell surface proteins (i.e. 'self' antigens) as being foreign and, thereby, initiates an immune response similar to the response to true foreign proteins [30]. This phenomenon is called an "auto-immune disorder." Below is an incomplete list of common auto-immune diseases. Since a dysfunctional immune system can, in theory, attack any cell type in the body and it can result in a very large variety of disease states, and a myriad of presenting symptoms within each disease. Some well-known entities here include: Type 1 Diabetes; Psoriasis; Systemic Lupus Erythematous; Multiple Sclerosis; Inflammatory Bowel Disease (i.e., Ulcerative Colitis and Crohn's Disease); and Rheumatoid Arthritis.

With this basic understanding of the immune system, it is easy to appreciate how deficiencies in the functions or responses to foreign threats can also result in significant disease states. For example, the Human Immunodeficiency Virus (HIV) is one of many viruses in which infection can result in a condition that impairs the ability of the human immune system to respond to certain types of infections [31]. Advanced or long-standing HIV infections, known as Acquired Immunodeficiency Syndrome (AIDS), can predispose to certain infections which can then be difficult to treat and even potentially life-threatening [32]. The most common cause of death in patients with advanced AIDS is often uncontrolled, overwhelming infection.

Fundamentally, the concept of "immunity" is based upon the inherent memory function of the immune system. The ability to recognize a repeat exposure and initiate a timely and effective response to attenuate the overall impact of an infection is a fundamental characteristic of the human immune system's ability to limit disease spread. The ability to efficiently attack a virus and limit its ability to replicate can be a cornerstone to not only reducing the impact of an infection on a patient, but more importantly, potentially limit transmission to other individuals (or a population). However, even with an intact immune system, immunity to an infection does not eliminate the potential for reinfection or disease spread—nor does it imply that the immune system's response to reinfection is less pathologic than the initial or re-infection itself. Furthermore, there are concerns and growing evidence to suggest that while certain diseases, such as certain strains of herpes viruses, can cause other pathologic conditions, such as certain malignancies, there are also concerns that auto-immune disease can be initiated as a consequence to the normal immune response to a "foreign antigen" that subsequently triggers a pathologic response to a "self antigen."

Fundamentals of Vaccines

Without a doubt, the development of vaccines against infectious diseases has been one of humanity's greatest achievements in terms of reducing the pain, suffering, and mortality associated with maladies that have plagued humans. The key principle behind a vaccine is to expose the immune system to an antigen that, while not inherently associated with an infectious disease, can elicit an immune memory response such that if the body is challenged with the complete infectious agent or antigen, it would be recognized and attacked in a manner that would attenuate any infectious complications [33]. Within the general microcosm of "mechanisms of vaccine action," there are several main types that will be discussed in this section.

Live attenuated vaccines: These types of vaccines involve inoculation with a "live" agent that has been biologically engineered to induce an appropriate immune response, but has been attenuated in a manner that reduces the risk of acute or severe infection [34]. While the risk of a true infection is minimal, it is not zero, and therefore "live vaccines" should not be avoided in patients who have impaired immune systems [35]. A major concern of this type of vaccine is that since the agent administered is still alive, in theory, it can evolve or mutate back into a pathogenic—and potentially more virulent—strain. While, by definition, the ability to replicate should be eliminated in the development process, such reactivation can occur [36, 37]. This is a well-known problem associated with the live oral polio vaccine. Examples of this include chicken pox (varicella), measles, mumps, and rubella. Of note, varicella zoster, the virus that causes Chicken Pox, is never completely eliminated by the human body and can be reactivated later in life, especially in patients with compromised immune systems, and cause complications in the form of zoster (Shingles), true reinfection is rare.

Killed/inactivated vaccines: Essentially, this type of vaccine is similar to the live vaccinate except that the infectious agent is "killed" during the development process—typically with either chemicals or heat. In theory, the ability to replicate and cause or transmit disease is eliminated, but it can still, as a function of the surface antigens, induce an appropriate immune memory response [38]. The polio vaccine is an example.

Inactivated toxin/toxoid: Certain types of infection are not caused directly by the bacteria or virus themselves, but the toxins that they produce and release into the body [39]. These types of vaccines are heat or chemically treated toxins that, while unable to cause disease, can still result in an appropriate immune response to attenuate potential risk for disease on exposure. The most commonly administered vaccine in this category is directed against the toxin produced by the bacteria *Clostridium tetani*—the toxin that causes tetanus [40].

Conjugate/subunit vaccine: These types of vaccines target specific surface proteins or structures that, while not inherently disease causing like the tetanus toxin, are uniquely associated with specific types of infectious agents [41, 42]. Because these types of vaccines are often very specific to certain bacteria or viruses, they can be extremely effective while also being very safe with regards to the risk of complications. Since these "subunit antigens" have no inherent reproductive or pathologic function, the risk of inducing disease is minimal. Conjugate vaccines work on the principle that a stronger and more robust immune response can be provoked by using more than one antigen associated with an infectious agent. Typically, cell surface components are linked with a carrier protein, which by definition is non-pathologic, that can produce an immune response. Vaccines directed against bacterial pneumococcal infections are an example of conjugate vaccines [43, 44].

Multiple/combination and booster vaccines: Some vaccines, such as measles, mumps, and rubella are administered together for convenience [45, 46]. Some vaccines require multiple staged (e.g., "booster") doses to maximize the immune response or to "boost" their impact [47].

Messenger RNA/nucleic acid vaccines: Among the most recent developments in our vaccine armamentarium is the arrival of messenger ribonucleic acid (mRNA) vaccines [48, 49]. Although not free of certain limitations, mRNA vaccines create a promise of 'vaccines on demand' where custom vaccinations can be made and implemented both quickly and efficiently, without the need for protracted incubations, risky deactivations, or synthesis of toxoids [50]. The science of mRNA vaccines is beyond the scope of this chapter, but the basic principle upon which they operate relies on the controlled introduction of mRNA material into the host and then host-based synthesis of the immune antigen within the host's own cells (without the risk of infection) [51–53].

The Concept of Herd Immunity

The basic principle behind "herd immunity" is that if sufficiently high proportion of the population have immunity (i.e., the herd) regardless of how acquired—vaccination, infection, or maternal-to-child transmission—the spread of the infection will be reduced [54]. Essentially, with diminished opportunities to infect, replicate, and spread due to the collective immunity of a population, the community impact of a bacterial or viral infection can be slowed or even stopped completely. While the exact percentage of a population (e.g., the herd) that needs to be immune to limit disease spread is a variable number based upon many factors, the concept is critical with regards to interventions aimed at preventing or limiting an epidemic or pandemic.

For example, the original estimated goal to achieve "herd immunity" for COVID-19 was approximately 70–75% of the population. This was based on data largely from the experience with the original COVID 19 strain from Wuhan, China, and may have evolved since then [55]. However, in December of 2020 four new strains of the virus were identified which had increased transmissibility. In Britain, a huge spike in cases was linked to the new strain, raising concern world-wide. The new strains impacted predictions to achieve "herd immunity" up to 80–85% of the population, per Dr. Jay Butler from the CDC [56]. Clearly, even with evolving herd immunity, disease transmission and potential reinfection is not eliminated [57]. The need to rapidly consider herd immunity at international/global level, rather than from a mostly local or national perspective has been illustrated by the concerns for spread of the original SARS, Ebola and other viruses in the early twenty-first century as international travel provides easy vectors for spread in a short period of time [58–60].

The Concept of a Novel Virus

The concept of a novel virus, while often used in the study of immunology and disease spread, gained substantial attention during the current Severe Acute Respiratory Syndrome Coronavirus 2 (SARS-CoV-2) pandemic associated with COVID-19 infections [2]. Essentially, a novel virus is one that has not been previously identified or recognized—often in the context of a specific species. Depending on the context, a novel virus can be known to exist in non-human animals and become novel once identified within a human transmission chain. There are countless viruses that have been shown to infect and cause complications in one species, but not another. However, once a virus starts to infect a species—such as humans—that has not been exposed to it previously, the lack of any immune memory from viral exposure, either at an individual or population level, can be catastrophic with regards to the inability to ward off potential infectious complications. The lack of any human prior exposure to SARS-CoV-2, much like any surprise military attack, resulted in humans (as individuals and as a population) being immunologically ill-prepared to fight off the infection and consequently was believed to explain, in part, the rapid and devastating spread of COVID-19 [61–63].

Immunity Records

The immune status of an individual is considered an essential part of their medical history and can be assessed, biologically, through several different approaches [64]. Each approach is based on different physiologic principles of what is known regarding the human immune system. The basis of recording immune status with regards to the exposure or infectious risks of a given individual, especially as applied to public health (or global health) initiatives and policies can be characterized by various strengths and limitations. In general, an immune record can consist of two key components:

1. *History of Infection*: As discussed above, with many infections—such as Chicken Pox—a previous infection and presumed normal immune response to that infection, reduces the risk of repeat infection and potential transmission.
   A history of infection can be: (a) self-reported; (b) documented as part of a patient's medical record; or (c) verified by testing for specific antibodies. Of importance, all of these modes of verification have potential limitations ranging from recall bias ("I think I had Chicken Pox when I was younger") to errors in the medical record interpretation (the "Flu" is a type of viral infection while "Influenza" is completely different type of bacterial infection) to the waning process in the immune memory system that might impact the body's ability to fight off a re-infection. Finally, as infectious agents mutate their antigen structures evolve over time, with "immune system memory" of previous infections no longer providing protection against another exposure.

For example, one might ask, "are we immune against smallpox?" After all, the eradication of smallpox (variola virus) has reportedly been accomplished; with the last documented case in 1977. Global containment initiatives, including a highly effective vaccine, were crucial in eradication [65, 66]. As a result of an effective global campaign against Smallpox, vaccination efforts in the United States were stopped in 1972. Still, if smallpox was to return, would it by definition again be a "novel virus?" Will our population have any "retained immunity?"

The waning of the immune system's memory response is well-known and the reason why certain vaccines, such as the Tetanus vaccine (see above), require booster shots periodically to maintain effective immunity. For many vaccines, the temporal immune response is poorly understood. While the development of memory response is often well-established for certain vaccines, the decay of that immunity is often more variable, complex, difficult to predict, and less under-stood on an individual level. For example, current evidence suggests that the SARS-CoV-2 mRNA-1273 vaccine (Moderna Inc, Cambridge, Massachusetts, USA) antibody response peaks at around 30 days and then slowly starts to decay. The peak titers and rate of decay was highly variable, and not just age-dependent, in the 34 people tested [67].

2. *History in immunization*: A history of vaccination—preferably documented and verified—is also another objective means to assist in documenting immunity against a potential infection. Since many vaccines are administered in childhood and required, at least in some parts of the world, prior to attending school, accurately maintained medical records can assist in providing proof [68, 69]. Access to a written medical record is not always possible (especially temporally remote childhood records for adults) and accuracy can be difficult to easily verify. Furthermore, as discussed above and as often seen with certain viral infections that are associated with high mutation rates (such as Influenza A—the virus that causes "the Flu"), vaccination against a particular infectious agent and antigen maybe not inherently convey protection against a newer or mutate strain [70]. Hence the need to undergo re-vaccination against "the Flu" each year.

3. *Objective testing*: Objective testing of immunity can be performed to demonstrate one's immunity. For example, blood concentration levels of antibodies directed against specific antigens can be measured and cut-off levels can be used to determine immunity. This is commonly used to determine objective immunity against Hepatitis B in a manner that is more accurate and sensitive than simply testing for the presence or absence of Hepatitis antibodies [71, 72]. Having said that, objective immunologic testing is not without challenges. For example, the Purified Protein Derivative (PPD), otherwise known as the Mantoux tuberculin skin test (TST) is commonly placed to detect infection with *Mycobacterium tuberculosis*—the agent that causes Tuberculosis (TB). A positive test can be used to demonstrate infection, but false positives can occur in patients with a history of vaccination—a point that is important since vaccination against TB is not com-monly administered in many parts of the world (including the United States) or because of antigen cross-reactivity with other types of mycobacterium that do not

cause TB [73, 74]. Similarly, false negative testing can occur in patients with pre-existing immune systems (including those with HIV who are also particularly prone to TB infections). There are other causes of inaccurate results from objective tests to determine immunity that illustrate the issues with using subjective or objective information to demonstrate the risks for disease transmission or acquisition. Also, it is important to fundamentally understand that just because a patient is immune to a disease, this finding does not eliminate the potential for subclinical or lesser infections or the ability to transmit an infection to another individual. At a basic level, immunity implies the body—or host—has developed a mechanism to minimize pathogen replication. In fact, it is this concept that serves as the basis for encouraging people to still wear masks to minimize the risk of spreading on becoming infected with COVID-19. This point is further emphasized, as previously mentioned, that the immune memory response to re-exposure or re-infection can wane over time - and in a manner is it sometimes unpredictable or poorly understood. For example, specifically related to SARS-CoV-2, there is some evidence that antibodies that developed in response to a known infection appear to persist for at least 6 months post-infection. This suggests that the risk for reinfection is low, but not zero, and unclear how long past 6 months antibodies persist to be effective against reinfection. Furthermore, in the setting of reinfection with existing and variable amounts of antibodies, it is unclear if there is an inverse relationship between antibodies levels or titers and recurrent disease severity [75]. To further complicate this concern is the uncertainty whether the decay in the memory response is different depending on whether it was obtained in response to an infection or a vaccine. These concepts are the logic behind why patients who had a previous documented infection should still get vaccinated and why vaccines are not 100% effective indefinitely and why, regardless of vaccine status and/or history of previous infection, people still adhere to appropriate precautions aimed at reducing disease spread [76].

As is clearly being demonstrated in the global race to develop a safe and effective vaccine against SARS-CoV-2, immunologic effectiveness and impact on disease severity and population spread can varying significantly. While preliminary Phase II and III clinical trials of initial COVID-19 vaccines under development across the world are promising, there is still much to learn regarding dosing, timing of booster shots, the impact on clinical variables and co-morbidities (such age, gender, weight, diabetes, heart/lung disease, renal disease, previous COVID infection, immune-modulating medications, etc.) on both short and long-term effectiveness [67, 77, 78]. Longer term (beyond 6 months) effectiveness of these vaccines combined with the evolving concerns regarding the durability of the human immune system response to COVID infection (and potential risk for re-infection, regardless of viral characteristics) are also evolving [79]. It must be emphasized that having received a vaccine does not always correlate with immunity and does not completely prevent disease or transmission—important concepts that must be considered when various "immunity passport" tools are being contemplated to help regulate social activity within the context of an outbreak or a pandemic.

Application of Blockchain Technology to Immunity Passports

As discussed above, the concept and need for "immunity passports" both represent an ideal application for the use of blockchain technologies [9]. Nevertheless, as we will discuss in subsequent paragraphs and sections of this chapter, there are numerous barriers to wide-spread use and acceptance of this approach, despite existing blockchain uses that cumulatively serve as an outstanding proof-of-principle that such applications can be successfully developed and deployed [8, 9]. Conceptually, an individual's vaccination and/or immunity history can be stored as a data element, encrypted of course, in a chain of blocks dedicated to storing such data. The inherent security and redundancy of the data ensure that the individual owner is the only one who has access to their immunity record. The built-in storage redundancies in the blockchain also ensure that the record is maintained privately, securely, and accurately—indefinitely and easily accessible. In theory, this sounds simple—but the practical applications and execution, as with everything else, especially in the context of a global community, remain the challenge and will be discussed below.

What Are the Data Elements that Need to Be Included?

If the data elements are considered a ledger to track immunity, then what are the specific data-fields that need to be recorded? For immunization records, typically type of vaccine, manufacturer, lot and serial numbers, date/location of administration are considered the minimum. Other variables may also be considered, such as more granular data regarding the anatomic location of vaccination (left vs right arm, etc.) and/or who administered the vaccine and which number in a sequence was given. Documentation of immunity can become much more complex and might include details regarding the test performed to verify immunity, date and time, test-type (plasma, salvia, tissue), manufacturer of the test, where the test was analyzed—and by whom, serial and lot numbers of reagents, and various government agency/health department safety and compliance tracking identifier.

Who Should Be Authorized to or Modify the Blockchain Record?

If the blockchain documenting immune status is to be considered an official record that can and will be used to allow participation in society, it is imperative that the accuracy and integrity of the data be as clear and pure as possible. Developing a process, with appropriate multi-factor authentication, any necessary redundancies, and safe-guards against fraudulent or inaccurate records while maintaining the necessary and desired privacy, will not be easy to implement. Simply expecting healthcare providers, who are already overburdened by administrative tasks and record keeping, to enter critical data in an accurate and timely fashion is an inherently unreasonable expectation. Third-party data entry systems must be trustworthy and free of many of the government, industry, and public systems that already reflect opportunities for misuse, corruption, and difficult to correct mistakes.

Who Owns the Private Key to Data?

As discussed above, access to encrypted blockchain data elements relies on access to both a public and private key. While public keys, by definition, can and should be widely available, access to the private keys reflects another concern. In theory, an individual should be the only one who has access to their private key and they should be able to control access to their corresponding data block. However, from a practical standpoint, is such an approach reasonable? Can and should others have access to private keys for valid reasons that might be potentially justifiable for a common good? Should government agencies, law enforcement, regulatory bodies, insurance companies, employers, parents, spouses, or healthcare providers have access to private keys, under a pre-specified set of legally transparent conditions? Entire systems must be established, on a global scale, to protect the privacy of the data—or, conversely, its utility might be limited as individuals might be reluctant to store or release their data out of concern that such data, regardless of the contents (i.e., immunity or lack thereof) might be used in a discriminatory or illegitimate manner.

Dealing with Loss of Private Key

Without a private key, the data elements cannot be accessed. Under the circumstances where private key is lost, how can the data be accessed in a timely and reliable manner? While redundant systems can, and probably should, be implemented, they must be built around the same requirements for accuracy, privacy, and accessibility as the primary blockchain. Even though a blockchain inherently contains redundancies and error-correcting mechanisms, if the private key is lost, access to the source data will be impossible (at least assuming modern computational capabilities versus the complexity of contemporary blockchain encryption methods).

Verification of Data Elements Versus Actual Immunity Status

Looking at the matter from global perspective, how can the records in an "immunity passport" (regardless of how stored) be relied upon to reflect true immunity. As discussed earlier in this chapter, true biologic "proof of immunity" can be very difficult and time-dependent. Even if a ledger can be established to accurately track vaccination history of patients against SARS-CoV-2, what will be the mechanism to address changes in immune status that naturally occurs from mutations, waning immune memory response, or the inherent variabilities in biologic responses that are often seen in patients with various degrees of immune system function (or dysfunction)? Using another infectious disease as an example, many countries will prevent border entry unless a traveler can document vaccination against Yellow Fever [80]. An acceptable form of documentation can be as simple as a folded piece of heavy paper with an official looking stamp and signature attesting to administration of a vaccine—hardly reliable and robust proof that such immunity in an individual exists. Nevertheless, the requirement for (and burden of proof) needs to be established and agreed upon in a manner that can accomplish the primary goal for why such "immunity passports" exist in the first place.

Demonstration of Required Data Elements by Individuals

With access to both a public and private key, how can a system be developed to ensure that an "immunity passport" and any corresponding data elements refer precisely to the user in question? Passports and travel visas often will contain pictures or biometric data that limit sharing of documents and/or make forgeries exceedingly difficult, but if an "immunity passport" is to be relied upon to limit the spread of a contagious disease, the burden of proof must be much higher than that of a regular "travel passport." Chain of custody of all data elements must be established and preserved at all times/levels. Simple pictures and multi-factor identification might not be sufficient. It is one thing for an individual to share their passwords and personal data to access bank accounts, but it is a completely different issue when such data can be shared to demonstrate immunity and allow for safe passage or participation in societal functions during a pandemic. More recently, two-factor authentication systems (i.e., passport and some verification of residence) are becoming more common.

Preventing Systemic Abuse

Paramount to any system to be effective as intended is for it to function appropriately and, in essence, as originally intended and/or designed. Without a doubt, given the potential implications for individuals and society, there are many opportunities for fraud, abuse, and criminal activities for personal and professional gain. End-to-end encryption, security, privacy, accuracy, integrity, and redundancy must be a fundamental cornerstone to whatever process is developed around any system using blockchain technology for immunity passports. Appropriate cross-checks must be included. While the technology inherently, by design, can minimize abuse, the processes that allow for data to enter the blockchain and subsequently used must consider malignant, criminal, and erroneous factors from the beginning. With every groundbreaking technology there is potential for unethical and/or outright criminal behavior.

Will Immunity Passports Be Effective?

A fundamental question regarding the use of "immunity passports" is focused on the concern whether vaccination programs will effectively prevent further disease spread. Without a doubt, there evidence that, regardless of the type of vaccine and disease, that vaccinations help with the control of the spread of disease across a population and may significantly attenuate the severity of disease within an individual [81]. Consequently, and without other factors in play, it is reasonable to assume that the issuance of "immunity passports" to all those vaccinated may provide an effective framework for wider reopening of the social and economic spheres of the society. At the same time, it is unlikely that vaccinations alone will be effective in completely controlling any outbreak or pandemic, and that other factors and interventions will be required as well [1]. For example, quicker and more accurate testing will continue to be critical, as well as the currently utilized non-pharmacological measures [7].

Who Should Pay for the Immunity Passport Framework Design and Implementation?

Within the microcosm of all the questions asked within this chapter, perhaps the most important and obvious questions must be asked at this time. Who will pay for the development and implementation of the "immunity passport" framework? How will data entry and verification occur? How about data storage and/or any data redundancy measures? How should training and education of users be conducted? What agency or organization will take ownership of the entire process and how will such an institution be funded—and in a manner that is transparent, private, and free to government or private industry agendas that might cloud the intent and purpose? While the costs for requiring "immunity passports" for international air travel can probably easily be incorporated into the costs of an airline ticket, how and who will fund the process that will be required to allow for a migrant worker across the world to visit their family in another country? Such systems must be equally accessible to all to prevent socio-economic, cultural, political, religious, gender, and other forms of discrimination. While costs, access to technology, and even vaccination availability might limit wide-spread adoption of "immunity passports," any actual implementations must be implemented in a manner that does not compromise or limit individual freedoms and basic human rights.

What Government, Group or Authority Should Determine Data Element Inclusion?

There are currently restrictions being considered for visitors to certain countries based on the specific COVID-19 immunization received. Examples may include the presence of specific viral mutation(s) or novel viruses, especially if the vaccine does not cover such mutation(s) or viral variants. Consequently, any "immunity passport" framework may require that a new data element is added to the "passport framework" from time to time. In addition, the World Health Organization (WHO) manages the internationally accepted standards for preventing the spread of diseases. The most recent publication, International Health (2005) outlines the agreed to legal and operational aspects of vaccines in international travel [82, 83]. This stems from the 1944 agreement that established the "Yellow Card"—a document mentioned earlier in the chapter and utilized for yellow fever control—which is currently recognized internationally. Presumably, the addition of a digital blockchain tool could be incorporated into suitable proposed WHO agreements in the future.

Management of Non-compliance

As with any policies that require vaccination prior to participation—like hospital employees being required to obtain annual influenza vaccinations as a condition of employment—there must be options for some degree of non-compliance or any "conscientious objectors" to the proposed vaccination and/or "immunity passport" regimen [84, 85]. Such policies, when appropriately implemented, do allow for individuals to "opt-out." However, such "opting-out" is typically associated with alternatives or consequences—such as limiting social interactions, mandatory mask-wearing, and some degree of objective verification of why they are refusing to be compliant (see below). Typically, objective verification is in the form of documented established religious exemptions or medical contraindications. Merely "not wanting" (for whatever subjective reason) is often inadequate. Unfortunately, especially with the rapidly evolving data regarding the safety, efficacy, and biologic interactions of the increasing number of vaccines that target SARS-CoV-2, the absolute and relative contraindications are in a state of flux [86].

From a social interaction perspective, if immunity or vaccination verification is to be mandated prior to a particular social or professional interaction, then some reasonable alternative options must be available. While it might be reasonable, to limit alternatives that might be considered "optional"—such as airline travel or attending concerts or sporting events—the legal consequences of such wide-spread policies will most likely be extremely controversial and extensively contested by multiple stakeholders, likely all levels. If an airline is going to restrict travel unless immunity is "appropriately or adequately" documented, then reasonable alternatives must be available. At least in the United States, such policies will most likely be closely scrutinized by the American Civil Liberties Union (ACLU) and must be compliant with the American with Disabilities Act [1]. How non-US industry and governments decide to address these topics will, no doubt, have unpredictable socio-economic and political consequences.

Despite various extensive challenges, there is growing interest in the development and broader implementation of "immunity passports." In addition, corporate leaders appear to support the concept of "immunity passport" implementation. For example, the Chief Executive Officer of Australia's Qantas Airlines, a company that has been severely impacted by various travel bans and global quarantines implemented in response to the COVID-19 pandemic, commented that significant "long-haul" (long-distance international flights) travel will not return until an effective vaccine is widely available and adopted. It was also implied that unless a traveler can document a "proof of a vaccine," in the form of an immunity or vaccination record, that international travel and entry into a specific country would be restricted (n.b. while there are a growing number of countries that are limiting entry, regardless of testing and immune status, there are significant legal concerns about preventing citizens from being able to return and enter into their own country) [86]. While these comments were inherently concerning in the context of the global implications on travel and trade, they do reflect an evolving consensus that proof of immunity might be required especially in the context of corporate and government liabilities for potentially propagating and making reasonable and appropriate efforts to mitigate against human-to-human infections. This concern is clearly highlighted in the death of an elderly passenger in December, 2020 from COVID-19, on a commercial airline flight from Orlando, Florida to Los Angeles, California. In the immediate aftermath, there was significant discussion regarding the obligations of airlines in general to screen and limit potentially infected patients from traveling. In addition, it is also unclear what the responsibilities, obligations, and liabilities are when a passenger is found to be infected and potentially actively infectious [87]. After all, if a traveler is known to be infected—how can they return home, especially if medical treatment is necessary and access is inherently complex and challenging. Obviously, the implications of these concerns will, extend beyond the COVID-19 pandemic. The least of which is the reality that people are already starting to counterfeit vaccination and testing result documentation to overcome the roadblocks of international travel [88].

While requiring vaccination prior to international travel and/or entry into foreign countries is not unreasonable, and potentially both practical and implementable, a larger debate is the issue of mandatory vaccination (or proof of immunity) before employees can return to work [89–91]. This is a concept supported by over 70% of 150 American corporate CEO's surveyed recently [92]. Currently, it is not unusual for healthcare employees (regardless of job description) to be required to demonstrate previously vaccination, infection, or immunity to common infections (i.e., chicken pox, hepatitis, tetanus, and annual flu vaccines). At least in the United States, the legal support for these practices is based upon the principle of a common good for society outweighs individual rights. Compulsory vaccination laws have been upheld by the Supreme Court of the United States with the provision that appropriate exclusions be available for "extreme cases" [93]. Despite many of these laws originating in the early twentieth century, they have been consistently upheld and even expanded to include requiring vaccination of students as a condition of enrollment [94]. However, we must acknowledge that the COVID-19 pandemic will most likely result in numerous policies and legal developments, regardless of scientific basis, that will challenge some of these legal precedents that are almost 100 years old.

A point of great importance that must be considered when discussing the topic of mandatory vaccination in the context of COVID-19 is that many (if not all) vaccines being deployed in early 2021 were approved under an Emergency Use Authorization (EUA) [95, 96]. At least in the United States, under the guidance of the Department of Health and Human Services, in working with the Federal Drug Administration (FDA), the level of safety and efficacy data is much lower than what it required for full regulatory approval (Biologics License Application - BLA). While requiring vaccination of an "approved" vaccine, which by definition has a much stringent efficacy, monitoring, and safety requirements is supported by many legal systems, the requirement for mandating vaccines only approved under an EUA is much more complicated and controversial legally and ethically [97].

Recognizing some of the numerous concerns of validating immunity and the lack of a common global format and trusted reporting system, the World Economic Forum and The Commons Project initiated the Common Trust Network. The purpose of this network, with support of key voluntary private and public institutions, was established to accomplish 3 major objectives [98]:

1. To empower individuals with digital access to their health information;
2. To make it easier for individuals to understand and comply with each destination's requirements, and
3. To help ensure that only verifiable lab results and vaccination records from trusted sources are presented for the purposes of cross-border travel and commerce.

To accomplish the above goals, participating organizations (including vaccination centers and laboratory testing sites) must agree to provide digital access to individuals using an open and globally-interoperated standard with verifiable credentials [99, 100]. While the specific digital tools and platforms to support this initiative were not specified, reference to support for Apple Health (Apple-based Operating Systems), CommonHealth (Google Android system), digital wallets, and appropriately verifiable printed QR codes. Despite these challenges, industry has already started developing passports focused on the consumer market [101]. Furthermore, the core principles behind the project include: openness and interoperability, transparency, neutrality, flexibility, inclusivity, sustainability, and privacy. Even though specifical applications (as of early 2021) are under development—such as the CommonPass app [102]—the technical aspects of data storage and access, taking into consideration the goals of the Common Trust Network appear to be an ideal application of blockchain technologies.

The application of blockchain technologies to immunity records—specifically for COVID-19—has been the focus of the IBM Digital Health Pass initiative [103]. In brief, this IBM initiative allows specific industries to partner with IBM to develop a unique digital platform, specific to the Industry (or corporate sponsor) to allow for trusted verification of immune status prior to individual participation. Several broad-based examples outlined by IBM in their promotional material included travel and transportation industries and sports/entertainment. As discussed previously, the basic premise is a joint IBM-Industry digital application, that conforms to CTN principles, in which an individual's immune credentials can be presented in real-time prior to engaging in social activities such as boarding an airplane or cruise ship, checking into a hotel, or attending conference, convention, or sporting event or concert. As case specific applications are driven by Industry (either as a single corporate initiative—like a single hotel chain developing their own specifications or requirements—or as a large-scale multi-corporate Industry consortium, like 'the travel thing that represents many global airlines), clearly there are concerns of fragmentation of applications, specifications, and standards. While a single digital application, based upon universal protocols and data elements, is desirable, the current approach suggests that multiple applications might be necessary. Given the current digital environment in which each corporation has their own branded applications, it is easy to envision a scenario (and maybe even integrated in these individual applications) in which separate applications are required to pass through airport security, board an airplane, aboard a cruise ship, and enter into each foreign port of call. While such fragmentation might be an initial approach based upon the existing foundations for individual credentials (boarding bases, reservation numbers, loyalty programs, and even digital-based visa), the goal should be directed towards a single set of standard verification data elements that are fully interoperable. An important consideration is that "immunity passport" applications be widely accessible and independent of socio-economic, religious, ethnic, and cultural backgrounds. The barriers to obtaining appropriate credentials, a digital platform, and the technology must adhere to the CTN principles of accessibility. Tools and initiatives that limit access to "luxury" or entertainment (corporate) events should not be applied to activities that might be considered essential human rights—such as education, employment, food, health care, and even basic transportation (government). The distinction between "necessary" and "luxury" activities can sometimes, culturally be blurred and varying across global societies; nevertheless they exist and must be considered. While such issues, including privacy, are not inherent to the use of blockchain in immunity passports, they are topics that must be considered.

With growing interest in controlling the spread of viral infections, especially COVID-19, and in response to evolving rules and regulations regarding travel and access, more and more institutions are requiring evidence of immunity, recovery, and vaccination. In response, much like the IBM digital health pass initiative, other groups are collaborating to develop digital tools. Microsoft and Oracle, have teamed up with industry leaders in the electronic medical space EPIC and Cerner, and the Mayo Clinic in Rochester, MN USA, along with other partners to form the Vaccination Credential Initiative [104]. While this collaboration is rapidly evolving with regards to having a functional solution, such large scale programs by Industry leaders demonstrate a growing global recognition of some of the issues that surround the need for verification of vaccination, exposure, and immunization records (and not just for COVID), access to timely and accurate information in a platform neutral manner (analog/paper/digital), and in a manner that is secure, safe, and is owned and controlled by the individual—not industry or government.

Despite the theoretical appeal of "immunity passports," the challenges of global implementation are bound to be difficult. The least of such challenges will be the acceptance of them as a useful tool in curbing the spread of disease. A study conducted at Duke University School of Medicine indicated that only half of physicians believe in their utility and 17% were uncertain. These findings were even more pronounced with less than 40% of US physicians supportive of passports [105]. Much like the reluctance of many segments of the population expressing concerns of early adoption of COVID-19 vaccines overall, without substantial support from healthcare providers, immunity passports might face similar roadblocks with wide-spread use.

Conclusions

The challenges of controlling the spread of highly contagious infections, as seen during the SARS-CoV-2 pandemic, introduced many concerns regarding the balance between social safety and individual freedoms. The discussions regarding the use of immunity passports to verify immune status and the ability to access countries, events and airline travel are a topic of discussion going forward. The use of a blockchain based "immunity passports" could help assure the integrity of the data, and avoid the ability to falsify information. However, there remain many societal issues regarding the use of such passports in a number of situations. In addition, there are access and technical issues that in the foreseeable future would limit it to a partial solution. In addition, as seen in Bitcoin, the permanent loss of information is possible if the private key is lost, and the remedies and solutions to this issue needs to be further evaluated for this solution to be implementable as a solution to proof of immunity.

References

1. Papadimos TJ et al (2020) COVID-19 blind spots: a consensus statement on the importance of competent political leadership and the need for public health cognizance. J Glob Infect Dis 12(4):167
2. Stawicki SP et al (2020) The 2019–2020 novel coronavirus (severe acute respiratory syndrome coronavirus 2) pandemic: a joint american college of academic international medicine-world academic council of emergency medicine multidisciplinary COVID-19 working group consensus paper. J Glob Infect Dis 12(2):47
3. Albrecht K (2006) Social intelligence: the new science of success. John Wiley & Sons
4. Bennett CJ (1992) Regulating privacy: data protection and public policy in Europe and the United States. Cornell University Press
5. Solove DJ (2013) HIPAA turns 10: analyzing the past, present, and future impact
6. Annas GJ (2003) HIPAA regulations-a new era of medical-record privacy? N Engl J Med 348(15):1486–1490
7. Stawicki SP et al (2020) Winning together: "C3–T2" updated COVID-19 infographic. J Emerg Trauma Shock 13(4):321–321
8. Stawicki SP et al (2019) Roadmap for the development of academic and medical applications of blockchain technology: joint statement from OPUS 12 global and litecoin cash foundation. J Emerg Trauma Shock 12(1):64
9. Stawicki SP, Firstenberg MS, Papadimos TJ (2018) What's new in academic medicine? Blockchain technology in health-care: bigger, better, fairer, faster, and leaner. Int J Acad Med 4(1):1
10. Paik H-Y et al (2019) Analysis of data management in blockchain-based systems: from architecture to governance. Ieee Access 7:186091–186107
11. Karafiloski E, Mishev A (2017) Blockchain solutions for big data challenges: a literature review. In: IEEE EUROCON 2017–17th international conference on smart technologies. IEEE
12. Hinkes AM (2019) Throw away the key, or the key holder? Coercive contempt for lost or forgotten cryptocurrency private keys, or obstinate holders. Northwest J Technol Intellect Prop 16(4):225
13. Judmayer A et al (2017) Blocks and chains: introduction to bitcoin, cryptocurrencies, and their consensus mechanisms. Synth Lect Inf Secur Priv Trust 9(1):1–123
14. Stevens H (2018) Hans Peter Luhn and the birth of the hashing algorithm. IEEE Spectr 55 (2):44–49
15. Wachira LW (2017) Error detection and correction on the credit card number using Luhn algorithm. COPAS, JKUAT
16. Li H et al (2013) An efficient merkle-tree-based authentication scheme for smart grid. IEEE Syst J 8(2):655–663
17. Yu M et al (2020) Coded merkle tree: solving data availability attacks in blockchains. In: International conference on financial cryptography and data security. Springer
18. Damgård IB (1989) A design principle for hash functions. In: Conference on the theory and application of cryptology. Springer
19. Tapscott D, Tapscott A (2017) How blockchain will change organizations. MIT Sloan Manag Rev 58(2):10

20. Donet JAD, Pérez-Sola C, Herrera-Joancomartí J (2014) The bitcoin P2P network. In: International conference on financial cryptography and data security. Springer
21. Sun JC, Ugolini S, Vivier E (2014) Immunological memory within the innate immune system. EMBO J 33(12):1295–1303
22. Goldrath AW, Bevan MJ (1999) Selecting and maintaining a diverse T-cell repertoire. Nature 402(6759):255–262
23. Dasgupta D (1993) An overview of artificial immune systems and their applications. In: Artificial immune systems and their applications, pp 3–21
24. Parham P (2014) The immune system. Garland Science
25. Amit A et al (1986) Three-dimensional structure of an antigen-antibody complex at 2.8 Å resolution. Science 233(4765):747–753
26. Mort M et al (2013) Vaccine safety basics: learning manual. World Health Organization
27. Liu M, Chen X (2021) COVID-19 basics and vaccine development with a Canadian perspective. Can J Microbiol 67(2):112–118
28. Rabadan R (2020) Understanding coronavirus. Cambridge University Press
29. Krishna M et al (2011) Diagnosis and management of hymenoptera venom allergy: British Society for Allergy and Clinical Immunology (BSACI) guidelines. Clin Exp Allergy 41 (9):1201–1220
30. Rose NR, Mackay IR (2006) The autoimmune diseases. Elsevier.
31. Hutchinson JF (2001) The biology and evolution of HIV. Annu Rev Anthropol 85–108
32. Weiss RA (1993) How does HIV cause AIDS? Science 260(5112):1273–1279
33. Zepp F (2016) Principles of vaccination. In: Vaccine design. Springer, pp 57–84
34. Minor PD (2015) Live attenuated vaccines: historical successes and current challenges. Virology 479:379–392
35. MAC of the Immune et al (2014) Recommendations for live viral and bacterial vaccines in immunodeficient patients and their close contacts. J Allergy Clin Immunol 133(4):961–966
36. Jeyaratnam J et al (2018) The safety of live-attenuated vaccines in patients using IL-1 or IL-6 blockade: an international survey. Pediatr Rheumatol 16(1):1–6
37. Williamson EM, Chahin S, Berger JR (2016) Vaccines in multiple sclerosis. Curr Neurol Neurosci Rep 16(4):36
38. Baxter D (2007) Active and passive immunity, vaccine types, excipients and licensing. Occup Med 57(8):552–556
39. Vetter V et al (2018) Understanding modern-day vaccines: what you need to know. Ann Med 50(2):110–120
40. Brook I (2008) Current concepts in the management of Clostridium tetani infection. Expert Rev Anti Infect Ther 6(3):327–336
41. Rappuoli R, Black S, Lambert PH (2011) Vaccine discovery and translation of new vaccine technology. Lancet 378(9788):360–368
42. Astronomo RD, Burton DR (2010) Carbohydrate vaccines: developing sweet solutions to sticky situations? Nat Rev Drug Discovery 9(4):308–324
43. Eskola J, Anttila M (1999) Pneumococcal conjugate vaccines. Pediatr Infect Dis J 18 (6):543–551
44. Lepoutre A et al (2015) Impact of the pneumococcal conjugate vaccines on invasive pneumococcal disease in France, 2001–2012. Vaccine 33(2):359–366
45. Farrington CP (1990) Modelling forces of infection for measles, mumps and rubella. Stat Med 9(8):953–967
46. Steele A et al (2010) Co-administration study in South African infants of a live-attenuated oral human rotavirus vaccine (RIX4414) and poliovirus vaccines. Vaccine 28(39):6542–6548
47. Leuridan E, Van Damme P (2011) Hepatitis B and the need for a booster dose. Clin Infect Dis 53(1):68–75
48. Pardi N et al (2018) mRNA vaccines—a new era in vaccinology. Nat Rev Drug Discov 17 (4):261

49. Jackson NA et al (2020) The promise of mRNA vaccines: a biotech and industrial perspective. npj Vaccines 5(1):1–6
50. Ulmer JB, Mansoura MK, Geall AJ (2015) Vaccines 'on demand': science fiction or a future reality. Expert Opin Drug Discov 10(2):101–106
51. Deering RP et al (2014) Nucleic acid vaccines: prospects for non-viral delivery of mRNA vaccines. Expert Opin Drug Deliv 11(6):885–899
52. Vogel AB et al (2018) Self-amplifying RNA vaccines give equivalent protection against influenza to mRNA vaccines but at much lower doses. Mol Ther 26(2):446–455
53. Zhang C et al (2019) Advances in mRNA vaccines for infectious diseases. Front Immunol 10:594
54. John TJ, Samuel R (2000) Herd immunity and herd effect: new insights and definitions. Eur J Epidemiol 16(7):601–606
55. Harrison C (2021) Future SARS-CoV-2 seasons–lessons to be learned from measles, rotavirus and influenza. Future
56. COVID_CDC_Team_Response et al (2020) Evidence for limited early spread of COVID-19 within the United States, January–February 2020. Morb Mortal Wkly Rep 69(22):680
57. Hall VJ et al (2020) Do antibody positive healthcare workers have lower SARS-CoV-2 infection rates than antibody negative healthcare workers? Large multi-centre prospective cohort study (the SIREN study), England: June to November 2020. medRxiv, p. 2021.01.13.21249642
58. Holmes KV (2003) SARS-associated coronavirus. N Engl J Med 348(20):1948–1951
59. Kalra S et al (2014) The emergence of ebola as a global health security threat: from 'lessons learned' to coordinated multilateral containment efforts. J Glob Infect Dis 6(4):164
60. Wojda TR et al (2015) The Ebola outbreak of 2014–2015: from coordinated multilateral action to effective disease containment, vaccine development, and beyond. J Glob Infect Dis 7(4):127
61. Chauhan V et al (2020) Novel coronavirus (COVID-19): leveraging telemedicine to optimize care while minimizing exposures and viral transmission. J Emerg Trauma Shock 13(1):20
62. Galwankar SC et al (2020) Management algorithm for subclinical hypoxemia in coronavirus disease-2019 patients: intercepting the "Silent Killer." J Emerg Trauma Shock 13(2):110
63. Sinha S et al (2020) Optimizing respiratory care in coronavirus disease-2019: a comprehensive, protocolized, evidence-based, algorithmic approach. Int J Crit Illn Inj Sci 10(2):56
64. Jarvis C (2018) Physical examination and health assessment-Canadian E-book. Elsevier Health Sciences
65. Fenner F (1982) Global eradication of smallpox. Rev Infect Dis 4(5):916–930
66. Henderson DA (2011) The eradication of smallpox–an overview of the past, present, and future. Vaccine 29:D7–D9
67. Widge AT et al (2021) Durability of responses after SARS-CoV-2 mRNA-1273 vaccination. N Engl J Med 384(1):80–82
68. Demicheli V et al (2013) Vaccines for measles, mumps and rubella in children. Evid Based Child Health Cochrane Rev J 8(6):2076–2238
69. Chen RT, Hibbs B (1998) Vaccine safety: current and future challenges. SLACK Incorporated Thorofare, NJ
70. Drake JW (1993) Rates of spontaneous mutation among RNA viruses. Proc Natl Acad Sci 90(9):4171–4175
71. Behzad-Behbahani A et al (2006) Anti-HBc & HBV-DNA detection in blood donors negative for hepatitis B virus surface antigen in reducing risk of transfusion associated HBV infection. Indian J Med Res 123(1):37
72. Chan HL-Y et al (2011) Hepatitis B surface antigen quantification: why and how to use it in 2011–a core group report. J Hepatol 55(5):1121–1131

73. Nayak S, Acharjya B (2012) Mantoux test and its interpretation. Indian Dermatol Online J 3 (1):2

74. Richeldi L (2006) An update on the diagnosis of tuberculosis infection. Am J Respir Crit Care Med 174(7):736–742

75. Lumley SF et al (2021) Antibody status and incidence of SARS-CoV-2 infection in health care workers. N Engl J Med 384(6):533–540

76. Paltiel AD et al (2021) Clinical outcomes of A COVID-19 vaccine: implementation over efficacy: study examines how definitions and thresholds of vaccine efficacy, coupled with different levels of implementation effectiveness and background epidemic severity, translate into outcomes. Health Affairs. https://doi.org/10.1377/hlthaff.2020.02054

77. Logunov DY et al (2021) Safety and efficacy of an rAd26 and rAd5 vector-based heterologous prime-boost COVID-19 vaccine: an interim analysis of a randomised controlled phase 3 trial in Russia. Lancet 397(10275):671–681

78. Xia S et al (2021) Safety and immunogenicity of an inactivated SARS-CoV-2 vaccine, BBIBP-CorV: a randomised, double-blind, placebo-controlled, phase 1/2 trial. Lancet Infect Dis 21(1):39–51

79. Dan JM et al (2021) Immunological memory to SARS-CoV-2 assessed for up to 8 months after infection. Science

80. Vanderslott S, Marks T (2021) Travel restrictions as a disease control measure: lessons from yellow fever. Glob Public Health 16(3):340–353

81. Caddy SL (2021) Few vaccines actually prevent infection–here's why that's not actually a problem, April 14, 2021. https://www.sciencealert.com/few-vaccines-actually-prevent-infection-here-s-why-that-s-not-a-problem-with-covid-19

82. Rodier G et al (2006) Implementing the international health regulations (2005) in Europe. Eurosurveillance 11(12):3–4

83. Le NK et al (2020) International health security: a summative assessment by ACAIM consensus group, in contemporary developments and perspectives in international health security-Volume 1. IntechOpen

84. Clarke S, Giubilini A, Walker MJ (2017) Conscientious objection to vaccination. Bioethics 31(3):155–161

85. Salmon DA, Siegel AW (2001) Religious and philosophical exemptions from vaccination requirements and lessons learned from conscientious objectors from conscription. Public Health Rep 116(4):289

86. Current_Affair (2020) Qantas boss says COVID-19 vaccination to be compulsory for international flights, April 14, 2021. https://9now.nine.com.au/a-current-affair/coronavirus-exclusive-the-compulsory-conditions-for-australians-to-travel-internationally-as-lockdowns-ease/e4bf2f6c-faab-46dd-8528-b7f8120ede2f

87. Sampson H (2020) Man who died following medical emergency on United flight had coronavirus, coroner says, April 14, 2021. https://www.washingtonpost.com/travel/2020/12/22/united-flight-passenger-death-covid/

88. Geiger G (2021) People are photoshopping COVID test results to bypass travel restrictions, April 14, 2021. https://www.vice.com/en/article/dy854a/people-are-photoshopping-covid-test-results-to-bypass-travel-restrictions

89. Mack A, Choffnes ER, Relman DA (2010) The domestic and international impacts of the 2009-H1N1 influenza a pandemic: global challenges, global solutions: workshop summary. National Academies Press

90. Zhang H et al (2010) Hub nodes inhibit the outbreak of epidemic under voluntary vaccination. New J Phys 12(2):023015

91. Ricciardi W, Boccia S, Siliquini R (2018) Moving towards compulsory vaccination: the Italian experience. Oxford University Press

92. Bigman D (2020) In poll, big-company CEOs say they're open to covid vaccine mandates, April 14, 2021. https://chiefexecutive.net/at-yale-summit-big-company-ceos-back-covid-vaccination-mandates-with-caveats/

93. Ehrenreich W (2008) Toward a twenty-first century jacobson v. massachusetts. Harv L Rev 121:1820, 1838–39
94. Buck_vs._Bell, 274 US 200 (1927). Craft, A. and Craft M. ibid, 2019.
95. Gee J (2021) First month of COVID-19 vaccine safety monitoring—United States, December 14, 2020–January 13, 2021. MMWR. Morb Mortal Wkly Rep 70
96. Oliver SE et al (2021) The advisory committee on immunization practices' interim recommendation for use of janssen COVID-19 vaccine—United States, February 2021. Morb Mortal Wkly Rep 70(9):329
97. Gostin LO, Salmon DA, Larson HJ (2021) Mandating COVID-19 vaccines. JAMA 325 (6):532–533
98. World_Economic_Forum (2021) Common trust network: covid action platform, April 14, 2021. https://www.weforum.org/projects/commonpass
99. W3C.org (2019) Verifiable credentials data model 1.0: expressing verifiable information on the web, April 14, 2021. https://www.w3.org/TR/vc-data-model/
100. Bender D, Sartipi K (2013) HL7 FHIR: an agile and RESTful approach to healthcare information exchange. In: Proceedings of the 26th IEEE international symposium on computer-based medical systems. IEEE
101. Ferdowsi S (2021) You can now get a COVID 'Passport' for $19.95: not everyone's happy about it, April 14, 2021. https://www.vice.com/en/article/bvx3nq/you-can-now-get-a-covid-passport-for-dollar1995
102. CommonPass.org (2021) CommonPass, April 14, 2021. https://commonpass.org/
103. IBM (2021) IBM digital health pass, April 14, 2021. https://www.ibm.com/products/digital-health-pass
104. MITRE_Corporation (2021) Vaccination credential initiative (VCI), April 14, 2021. https://vci.org/
105. Doraiswamy PM et al (2020) Are we ready for COVID-19's Golden Passport? Insights from a Global Physician Survey. medRxiv

Digital Identity, Computational Reliabilism, and the Future of IOMT: Epistemic Reasoning and the Role of Blockchain in Removing Human Tampering from Pharmacovigilance Decision Making

7

Mateusz Plaza, Sean Batzel, Thomas Wojda, and M. M. Alcaro

Tali sono tutte le cose vere, doppo che son trovete; ma il punto sta nel saperle trovare.

—Galileo Galilei

Measure what is measurable, and make measurable what is not so.

—Antoine-Augustin Cournot and Thomas-Henri Martin

Abstract

This chapter advocates for the use of on-chain digital identities to eliminate human tampering from pharmacovigilance decision making, thereby justifying the reliability of blockchain for medical and pharmaceutical technologies. Through the use of the hash function (SHA256) and Proof of Work, blockchain allows for IOMT digital identities that are authentic, accurate, and reliable. We draw upon Juan Durán's work on computational reliance in computer

M. Plaza (✉)
Philadelphia College of Osteopathic Medicine, 4170 City Ave, Philadelphia, PA 19131, USA
e-mail: mp7324@pcom.edu

S. Batzel
Drexel University, 3141 Chestnut Street, Philadelphia, PA 19104, USA
e-mail: stb69@drexel.edu

T. Wojda
University of Pittsburgh Medical Center, Pittsburgh, USA
e-mail: wojdatr@upmc.edu

M. M. Alcaro
Rutgers University, 510 George Street, New Brunswick, NJ 08901, USA
e-mail: mma235@scarletmail.rutgers.edu

simulations and algorithms, as well as Sanford Goldberg's social epistemological work on diffuse reliance, to create our own concept– blockchain computational reliabilism (BCR)– which justifies the reliability of on-chain digital identity through three form of BCR, including appeal to expertise, algorithmic competence, and measurement robustness. Ensuring the integrity of on-chain digital identities by excluding the possibility of human tampering thus paves the way for a possible solution to the decision making problems that pharmacovigilance scientists currently face.

Keywords

Blockchain · Epistemology · Digital identity · Pharmacovigilance · Decision making · Reliabilism · Philosophy of science · Medicine · Metrology · IOMT · Bitcoin · Proof of Work · Algorithm · Epistemic reasoning

Introduction

On September 20, 2020 the World Health Organization (WHO) announced that the world was experiencing an "infodemic." Their resolution emphasized that overwhelming misinformation and disinformation was undermining the dissemination of information grounded in science and evidence; the consequence was ineffective public health measures. The WHO made a public request for better digital infrastructures that support healthier information flows [1].

Today, pharmacovigilance decision makers (PVDM) face an enormous challenge. While pharmacovigilance relies on science and evidence to detect, assess, understand, and prevent patients from being harmed by undiscovered or undesirable adverse reactions (ADR), pharmacovigilance scientists are already working in resource-constrained conditions [2]. Research on information overload in organizations notes that each organization has an "information processing capacity" (IPC) [3]. With millions of Internet of Medical Things (IOMT) and their human users generating an ever-increasing amount of data, pharmacovigilance decision makers, already at their IPC, face the additional challenge of human tampering, which encompasses everything from innocent transcription errors to malignant hacks. The overwhelming amount of data combined with data hacks and breaches has left pharmacovigilance decision makers caught in what conflict prevention decision makers call "the wicked problem." A term frequently used by early-warning signaling scholars, "the wicked problem" refers to the challenge of making a well-informed decision due to an incomplete knowledge base coupled with a lack of an evaluation standard. The infodemic and its resulting wicked problem will undoubtedly plague PVDM in the decade to come, when IOMT device usage is anticipated to increase decision making complexity by 70% and result in the influx of even more data [4]. However, steps can, and must, be taken today to mitigate and manage the wicked problem that PVDM face by eliminating the possibility for human tampering. For this solution, we turn to blockchain technology; specifically, the usage of on-chain digital identity for IOMT devices.

This essay advocates for the use of on-chain digital identities to eliminate human tampering from the process of pharmacovigilance decision making, thereby justifying the reliability of blockchain for medical and pharmaceutical technologies. To do so, we draw upon interdisciplinary scholarship from such diverse fields as social epistemology, conflict prevention, philosophy of science, digital forensics, and computer-based ethics.

In 2014, Juan Durán drew upon Alvin Goldman's work on process reliabilism in order to justify scientific reliance on computer simulations and algorithms. Durán leveraged Goldman's concept of "process reliabilism," an epistemic justification stating that a process is more likely to continue behaving as it always has than to stop behaving in that way [5, 6]. In 2018, Durán formalized a computer-focused version of process reliabilism called "computational reliabilism." Durán uses computational reliabilism to argue for the justification of computer simulations in the context of scientific decision making and medical ethics [7, 8]. In this past year (2020) he has turned to how computational reliabilism might help us better rely upon medical AI and decision making [9]. Also inspired by Goldman's work, but coming from the discipline of social epistemology, Sanford Goldberg ushered the problem of process reliabilism into a social epistemological context, coining the phrase "diffuse epistemic reliance" in order to talk about how we can rely on multiple people's cognitive processes in order to ascertain if information is trustworthy [10, 11].

The algorithm in blockchain's Proof of Work algorithm—an example of a computational process—justifies the use of Durán's computational reliabilism to verify that information, but the decentralized nature of the blockchain network adds a layer of complexity; for, where Durán's work on computer simulation and centralized algorithms deals with a single entity in control, blockchain relies on multiple nodes to run its network. This is where Goldberg's social epistemological framework is useful. If we think of the blockchain network's nodes as peers (essentially, people), we begin to see that in relying on miners to run the blockchain network, we are, as Goldberg says, relying on others. In simultaneously confronting the problems of algorithm-based reliability and diffuse reliance, blockchain technology addresses–and indeed, seems to solve–one of the problems facing pharmacovigilance decision makers today: human tampering in the digital identification of IOMT devices.

An on-chain digital identity ensures that no human tampering of the manufacturer's given IOMT digital identity has occurred; it does this by providing evidence that the digital identity is authentic (having the proper provenance), accurate (having a verifiable unbroken chain of custody), and reliable (producing convincing reason for justified belief). The evidence that on-chain digital identity provides is *accurate* in large part because the hash function (SHA256) enables the on-chain identity to have evidential provenance from the manufacturer. It is *authentic* because the digital signature and public key cryptography prove ownership of the original data input at the digital identity's genesis. The evidence is *reliable* because the Proof of Work (PoW) process allows pharmacovigilance decisionmakers to justify their reliance on on-chain identity through blockchain computational relia- bilism in the form of appeals to expertise, algorithmic competence, and measure- ment robustness. An on-chain identity secured by blockchain-based cryptography and PoW algorithm, therefore, allows pharmacovigilance decision makers to jus- tifiably exclude the presence of human tampering with an IOMT's digital identity, thus paving the way for a solution to the wicked problem that PVDM currently face.

In order to resolve the wicked problem facing PVDM, we must ensure that IOMT digital identity is both accurate and authentic; this can only be done by removing the human element and delegating these tasks to blockchain-based ID proofing. We ensure that this digital identity remains free of human tampering through the PoW algorithm, which is itself computationally reliable for many reasons, foremost among them because of expertise, algorithmic competence, and measurement robustness: tools we already use to ensure that scientific decision making is reliable.

Digital Identification and Its Challenges

The first step in our analysis is to establish a firm understanding of what digital identity entails. The National Institute of Science and Technology (NIST) describes the process of providing IOMT devices with a digital identity as the "ID Proofing" process, where ID Proofing is the process that "establishes that a subject is who they claim to be" [12]. In this case, the "subject" is the physical IOMT device. This physical IOMT device engages in online transactions through its online represen- tation; the digital identity represents the interactions a physical IOMT device has with the networked technology sphere. The concept of "uniqueness" is what allows for precise measurements and analyses of the digital identity. By "unique" what we mean is "discrete;" digital identity is something that can be counted as an individual entity. To ensure a digital identity is discrete, it should have a 1:1 correspondence to the physical IOMT device [13]. By ensuring a 1:1 correspondence, the digital representation, like the physical IOMT device, is discrete; therefore, a 1:1 corre- spondence allows an IOMT device to have the discreteness it needs to be scien- tifically counted. In order to create a digital identity, the NIST provides a mechanism called ID Proofing, which verifies that the physical IOMT device and digital representation have a 1:1 correspondence [14].

An IOMT digital identity is important because it enables pharmacovigilance systems makers to aggregate, collect, and analyze safety information coming from a specific physical IOMT device, including data like cybersecurity audit logs [15]; IOMT device manufacturing and distributing history [16]; and pharmaceutical drug manufacturing and distribution history [17, 18]. By harmonizing data sources in this way, an IOMT digital identity becomes a reference point for pharmacovigilance decision makers to find evidence about the IOMT device (like audit logs of an IOMT device's access controls).

If an IOMT digital identity is comprised in such a way that it no longer represents the IOMT device, there is no way for pharmacovigilance scientists to determine whether an IOMT device is creating danger to patients [19]. A recent study into possible cyberthreats to life-sustaining cardiac IOMT devices discovered 11 cyberattack scenarios. In each of these scenarios, the best-case scenario was massive data breach and incomplete data evidence; the worst-case scenario was patient death due to malicious cyberattack [20]. If an IOMT's digital identity cannot authenticate a patient into a hospital's database, then there is no way for physicians to monitor a patient's health or react to any sudden changes in patient status. Some cyberattacks can both inactivate an IOMT's link to healthcare and pharmacovigilance data systems, thus putting the patient using the IOMT device at an increased risk of death; this is particularly true for patients relying on IOMTs for life-saving medical treatments, such as cardiac or diabetic support [21].

Yet the existence of digital identity alone is not enough to ensure that IOMT device identity remains both accurate and authentic. A significant threat to the integrity of digital identity is human tampering, which falls under two major categories: error and malicious action. Repeat ID Proofing by human agents during the manufacturing and distribution process can lead to human error (and even subsequent fraud) in verifying the correct physical device with the respective digital representation.

Human tampering in the form of human ID Proofing of an IOMT device identity could lead to errors in input. In one study, researchers found human ID Proofing to result in only 31% accuracy, meaning only 31% of digital identities remained linked to their corresponding physical item [22]. This is also a problem in pharmaceutical drug counterfeiting. It is common for humans to process pharmaceutical medication quantities and prescriptions by ID Proofing manually. Malicious actors take advantage of this in order to commit fraud by intentionally labeling a physical drug with the wrong digital identity so as to make the drug more desirable for customers. The issue of drug counterfeiting is a serious issue worldwide, with research estimating that around 10% of the world drug supply is counterfeit [23, 24]. Recently, Pfizer announced there were counterfeit versions of their COVID 19 vaccine, which could obviously have damaging effects on global health [25].

Furthermore, certain network cyberattacks, like man-in-the-middle (MIM) attacks, can separate the IOMT digital representation from the IOMT physical device through identity impersonation, theft, and eavesdropping. In the case of human tampering by malicious action, the most common form comes from cyberattacks against the network layer. Network layer cyberattacks "steal" digital identities, allowing for unauthorized usage of that digital identity. Since it is an IOMT device's network layer that allows the device to communicate through network infrastructure (like the internet), common cyberattacks target the IOMT device's network layer, including traffic analysis attacks, selective forwarding attacks, sinkhole attacks, botnet attacks, hello-flood attacks, and man-in-the-middle attacks. In the case of MIM, malicious actors compromise both the digital identity and information connected to the digital identity. Because in MIM malicious actors compromise the 1:1 correspondence between the digital identity and physical device by taking control of the digital identity, impersonating the IOMT's digital identity allows malicious actors to eavesdrop on communications online, leak data to the public, or change data content [26].

Unfortunately, cyberattacks are an all-too-common occurrence. Internet users frequently have poor cybersecurity practicesPractice which, in the context of IOMT, make the digitalDigital identityIdentity an easy target for cyberattacks [19]. Third-party technology vendors for pharmacovigilance systems might also be affected. One study shows that 56% of companies using third-party digital services have had their third-party service provider compromised by cybersecurity breaches [27]. The underlying cause of user or third-party cyberattacks can be traced to some form of human error; research shows that 95% of cybersecurity breaches are caused by human error providing malicious actors with an easy target of attack [28].

Ensuring Accuracy and Authenticity

We have mentioned the importance of digital identity's being both authentic and accurate in order to keep it safe from cyberattacks. Pharmacovigilance scientists can assess an IOMT digital identity's *accuracy* by seeing if the digital identity was created by the manufacturer. An IOMT digital identity is said to be *authentic* if it is one given to the device by the manufacturer. Since the manufacturer is the genesis of the IOMT digital identity and is trustworthy, an authentic digital identity is an accurate digital identity.

Scientists measure accuracy by comparing experimental results with a defined standard of measurement [29]. One can measure IOMT digital identities using the physical IOMT device as a standard; specifically, an IOMT digital identity is accurate if it has a 1:1 correspondence with an underlying IOMT physical device. Assuming the genesis of an IOMT's digital identity occurs at IOMT manufacturing ID Proofing, and assuming the manufacturer is trustworthy, one can see the manufacturer's ID Proofing process as creating an accurate IOMT digital identity [30].

But how can PVDM ensure that a device is both accurate and authentic? While human tampering like MIM disrupts the intelligibility of an IOMT digital identity, the disruption is not apparent; instead, human tampering like MIM is nefarious and hidden. From the perspective of the pharmacovigilance scientist, a malicious actor impersonating an IOMT device will seem the same as a genuine IOMT device, since both cases use the IOMT digital identity, which is what the scientist relies on for scientific analysis. The consequence is that a pharmacovigilance decision maker does not have a standard of evaluation to indicate whether an IOMT digital identity has been compromised; however, she still must make a decision in order to fulfill her duties to her patients. This state of being unable to make a decision due to an apparent lack of evaluative standards is known as a "wicked problem" [31]. In order to resolve this problem, PVDM must find a way to ensure that their digital identification is both accurate and authentic. This is where blockchain technology, specifically on-chain identity, comes in.

Blockchain to the Rescue

The term "blockchain technology" is used in various industries. As a general data technology class, people might recognize the hallmark values that blockchains provide for data: immutability, decentralization, distribution, encryption, and tokenization [32]. Despite these general value propositions, there is a great amount of diversity among blockchains; there are hundreds, if not thousands, of blockchain protocols, each with a unique approach to supporting those hallmark value propositions. Our essay focuses specifically on Bitcoin's protocol, which is the most well-known protocol due to its success with cryptocurrency investors. Created by the anonymous Satoshi Nakamoto, Bitcoin's technology leverages two cryptographic methodologies to ensure the completeness of digital identity and its respective online transactions: a SHA256 hash function and Proof of Work (PoW) consensus algorithm.

SHA 256 and PoW protect the discreteness—and thus 1:1 correspondence—of IOMT digital identities; in so doing, blockchain technology can protect digital identity's evidential provenance. Additionally, PoW ensures that no human can tamper with an IOMT's digital identity by utilizing the SHA256 as a measurement instrument. The way PoW does this is by ensuring each IOMT digital identity is immutable, which is to say the IOMT digital identity is unchangeable over time. In turn, PoW provides decision makers with reasons to believe an on-chain identity has not been subject to human tampering. Bitcoin's SHA256, public-key cryptography, and cryptographic digital signatures thus provide pharmacovigilance scientists with an authentic and accurate IOMT digital identity.

Public-key cryptography allows for encrypted communication over a computer network. Each user creates their own public and private key pair, sharing their respective public keys to everyone else using the computer network. To send a secure message, a user encrypts her message using another user's public key and sends the message to him. The recipient then decrypts the message using his own private key [33, 34].

A cryptographic digital signature's basic purpose is to prove ownership of public keys without disclosing private keys; a user digitally signs their public key, their digital signature proves the public key belongs to the owner of the private key, without disclosing the private key [33, 34].

The Hash Function: SHA256

SHA256 is a hash function whose purpose is to convert arbitrary data inputs into 256-bit string outputs. A small change in data input results in significant differences in outputs. Bitcoin leverages SHA256 to make it computationally infeasible to find:

1. the input data from the output hash
2. another input with the same hash value
3. two data input points that result in the same hash value

SHA256 employs a cryptographic process that ensures each hash is unique, taking an input and converting it into a unique hash. In the case of the IOMT digital identity, a new block is created by the inputs of the previous block's hash + the digital identity. At this point, the new hash is a unique object that connects the IOMT digital identity data to the previous block's hash. This previous block contains its unique IOMT digital identity data as well as the hash of the previous block, and so on. There is a chain of blocks that depend on each other (hence the name "blockchain"). If there is a change to the previous block, then there is a change to all the following blocks. This ensures that any change to on-chain data is immediately noticeable, because it changes the content of the consequent blocks on the ledger. When a digital identity is thus added to the blockchain via the SHA256 function, it is a unique mathematical object.

The Proof of Work (PoW) Algorithm

Proof of Work adds a third component called a "nonce" to this hash; "nonce" stands for "number used only once." This nonce gets added with the previous hash and the digital identity to create a unique hash. The PoW algorithm then arbitrarily adds a series of zeros at the start of the hash called "difficulty" [35]. PoW then challenges all the computers to use computational power to discover the nonce that would combine with the previous block's hash and the digital identity to create the hash with a matching number of leading zeroes (called the "difficulty setting"). PoW transmits this challenge to the entire network and all the computers start systematically testing every possible solution, which would be the nonce that corresponds to the hash that has a set number of zeros at the start (its difficulty) and which is the resulting hash of the previous block's hash combined with the digital identity. Eventually one of the nodes in the network finds the right nonce for the right hash; when this occurs, we say the node has "mined" a block. (It is also for this reason that these nodes are called "miners.") The node has put in computational power to systematically generate every possible nonce, until the right nonce is found commensurate to the hash that is created by the previous block's hash, the new digital identity and the arbitrary zeroes at the start of this hash.

When a node (or miner) discovers the correct nonce-hash pair, the node transmits the solution to all the other nodes in the network. The other nodes check the miner's answer by comparing it to their copy of the ledger. Since the other nodes have an entire copy of the ledger, they can create the hash with the same number of zeroes at the start. Once miners discover the correct nonce other miners can instantly verify the solution against the desired hash, which they can create by using their ledger; this ensures that verifying the solution is easier than finding the solution. Each of these nodes can check the miner's answer by using their ledger. The other nodes take the previous hash, the new digital identity, and the proposed nonce, hash it, and see if it results in the right hash, which is one with the right number of zeroes at the start. If the proposed nonce generates the right hash, then it is accepted to the active ledger. Each of the nodes in the network do this, allowing the correct answer to propagate throughout the network.

Computational Reliabilism

We suggest that pharmacovigilance decision makers could use "computational reliabilism" to justify their reliance on the authority of Proof of Work. Here, reliabilism refers to an epistemic principle that seeks to explain knowledge or justification in terms of "truth-conduciveness" of the process by which an individual forms a true belief [6]. In layman's terms, we call a process *reliable* if it provides more reason for us to arrive at a true outcome than a false one. Going beyond the belief-forming process that Goldman called "process reliabilism," computational reliabilism states that "claims about knowledge need to be located within a theoretical framework that properly articulates these sources and supplies a justification of the reliability of the computer simulation along with reasons to believe in their results" [8]. It's important to note a key distinction here; while process reliabilism doesn't include a justificatory chain, for scientific study, it is important to have reasons to choose one course of action over another, and have a way of scientifically verifying the reason for choosing that course of action. Computational reliabilism, then, allows for scientists to apply scientific methods to evaluate their own justifications of computer simulations or, in this case, algorithms [9]. Taking Durán's work a step further, a blockchain-specific version of computational reliabilism, (what we are calling "blockchain computational reliabilism" or "BCR") would state:

> (BCR): The probability that the next set of results of a reliable consensus algorithm is trustworthy is greater than the probability that the next set of results is trustworthy given that the first set was produced by an unreliable process by mere luck.

BCR has many sources by which it justifies the results of PoW, an algorithm. Among these sources, we wish to highlight expertise (both tried and true methods as well as individual academic authorities); algorithmic competence (a term coined by Plaza to indicate the skill of the algorithm to achieve relevant information furthering practical information goals of the community); and measurement robustness (a convergence of evidence caused by decentralized nodes, seen as a measurement system).

While there are those who are suspicious of blockchain technologies, in using BCR to justify our reliance on the PoW algorithm, we are not deviating from the current paradigmatic standard typically employed by pharmacovigilance decision makers, or indeed, members of the scientific community at large [35]. Standard reasons for justifying the reliability of current scientific findings frequently rely upon an appeal to previous scientific authorities (expertise); socially normative competence of a researcher in her profession (congruent to what we call algorithmic competence); and proper instrument calibration (measurement robustness). These sources of BCR are treated in detail below.

Expertise: History of Theoretical Development

In speaking of "expertise," we refer to both recorded methodological progress of a scientific focus and the individual authorities who create and develop them. Any base of scientific knowledge is accumulated and built upon through years of study and trial and error, resulting in the perpetuation of only those with the most explicatory force [36]. Thus one source of reliability for a blockchain's consensus algorithm comes from the history of the protocol's development specifically, the failures and consequent successes of a consensus algorithm's implementations justify the reliability of the consensus algorithm [8]. This source of reliability draws its justificatory power from the history of science and importantly from the history of a particular scientific object's investigations. In the case of a blockchain consensus algorithm's history of development, there are years of improvement and refinement of the science and engineering behind the blockchain consensus algorithm. As a consensus algorithm develops further, the methodologies to build the consensus algorithm develop "techniques are improved upon, reconfigured, and radically revised when the technology changes or a new method is envisaged" [8]. A consensus algorithm, then, does not improve independently of the scientific methodologies used to research and develop it; therefore, pharmacovigilance decision makers can look at the history of a blockchain consensus algorithm's development to see the way in which the scientists developed it.

Bitcoin's PoW consensus algorithm has a public record of all its developments. One place where this is readily observable is on Bitcoin's GitHub repository. By looking through Bitcoin's GitHub, decision makers can see a robust and diverse array of discussions and analyses of various methodological and empirical investigations into the nature of the Bitcoin ledger, as well as its consensus algorithm's development. Decision makers can quickly see that Bitcoin's scientific community abides by high computer engineering and scientific standards, keeping track of experiments and results; most importantly, there is an improvement of the science as time progresses.

An example exemplifies this point best. On February 13, 2011 a Bitcoin GitHub user called "kasperhartwich" posted an issue called "Specify location for wallet.dat file #68." This issue was a proposal to improve some aspects of Bitcoin's technology. The rest of the Bitcoin community responded with various ideas and engineering solutions to tackle this request. In the end, the issue gathered 21 comments with a variety of engineering and scientific approaches to solve the issue the original user posted. In the end, after thorough review, the Bitcoin development team implemented the update to Bitcoin's networking technology. After the issue was resolved, the Bitcoin community closed the issue and left a record of the issue in GitHub. At this point, this issue, its consequent discussion, and its successful implantation as a Bitcoin update represents one part of a diverse and robust history of Bitcoin's development. GitHub provides the Bitcoin community with ways to label certain scientific proposals, utilizing labels like "Brainstorming," "Feature," "Idea," "Bug," "Build System."

Blockchain technologies rely on open source and open science development strategies to increase the diversity of approaches to blockchain science. This means consensus algorithms such as Bitcoin's PoW have years of records of the consensus algorithm's scientific work; consequently, this history log becomes a source of reliability for the PoW consensus algorithms. The GitHub based scientific history log would show pharmacovigilance decision makers that there is a firm knowledge base and community of experts developing, creating, and refining the best possible scientific approaches to blockchain consensus algorithms. In total, therefore, a history of scientific research and development of Bitcoin supports blockchain computational reliabilism because it is more likely that the history of Bitcoin technology's development is based in a reliable methodological evolution than it is that this methodology appeared by pure luck [37].

Expertise: Expert Authorities

As we have established, blockchain consensus algorithms have a scientific community that experiments and develops methodologies and approaches to improving blockchain consensus algorithms (and other components of the blockchain's technology); the improvement of blockchain science methodologies occurs in parallel to the improvement of the blockchain technology itself. This shows blockchain science has a defined and growing research focus in academic work, including emerging experts on blockchain technology. This represents a standardization of blockchain expertise, leading to the establishment of blockchain expert reliability.

Pharmacovigilance decision makers can observe the formalization of blockchain expertise in the open source, open science community, as well as in traditional academic peer-review settings. Although GitHub relies on open source and open-source work that theoretically anyone could participate in, the actual ability to contribute to blockchain algorithms and other parts of blockchain science is restricted to a vetted epistemic community, in turn ensuring that GitHub's methodological and empirical work on blockchain consensus algorithms is carried out by blockchain experts [38]. The open science, open source community—such as GitHub's Bitcoin community—has a peer-review process and self-selection process that ensures blockchain experts contribute and come to scientific consensus on the best blockchain science practice, methodology, and standards [39].

There is also a formalization of blockchain expertise in traditional academic entities, evidenced by a rise in bibliometric analyses. A glance at bibliometric analyses from 2021 reveals the scope and breadth of blockchain experts currently at work. Additionally, 2021 bibliographic analysis of blockchain research provides an estimate of academic blockchain articles published between 2013–2020; the top five subjects are their respective research article quantity are computer science (3839 articles), electrical and electronic engineering (1393 articles), telecommunications (1037 articles), energy fuels (116 articles), and industrial engineering (113 articles) [40]. Increasingly, traditional academic institutions are focusing their resources on exploring and understanding blockchain technology. Furthermore, blockchain experts are emerging in such diverse fields as security, transportation, logistics, and finance.

A growing body of blockchain experts ensures the maintenance of high standards of research and development of blockchain science; critically, these experts are involved in the practical implementation of blockchain consensus algorithms through open science and open-source work. Consequently, expert knowledge becomes a source of reliability for PoW. Since experts maintain standards with the intention of creating systematic and reliable methodologies of scientific reasoning, it helps support a blockchain computational reliabilist justification of the PoW consensus algorithm; that is, experts are more likely to develop expertise that expand and innovate standards if PoW were a reliable algorithm, then if experts would expand their expertise by pure luck.

Algorithmic Competence (Virtue Epistemology)

In John Greco's work *The Transmission of Knowledge,* computer programming is called a "hinge commitment." Hinge commitments are a subtype of procedural knowledge that constitute the successful generation and transmission of knowledge. Greco writes about these commitments constituting a human being's cognitive hinge commitments. According to him, these hinge commitments constitute competent cognitive processing in the form of the generation and transmission of knowledge. Greco does not, however, spend any time extending his work into computational reliabilism or blockchain computational reliabilism, as this essay does. That being said, he does provide enough analysis to *justify* such an extension. Greco writes that one can see computer programming is analogous to the internalization of rules by human cognitive processes [41]. He also writes that computer programming that is hardwired is analogous to the "built in" part of the human cognitive process. Greco is, however, unclear on whether this "built in" process pertains to the brain or genetics. Either way, there is enough to warrant exploration of the way in which Greco's virtue epistemological defense of an information economy relates to computational reliabilism in blockchain technology.

By applying Greco's concept of competence to BCR, we can justify the BCR of PoW through the concept of "algorithmic competence." By viewing the PoW consensus algorithm through the lens of an information economy, then one can see that a PoW consensus algorithm reliably protects an on-chain IOMT digital identity from human tampering because the PoW consensus algorithm is competent at producing knowledge of a tamper-free IOMT digital identity [41].

Consider how the PoW consensus algorithm secures and protects Bitcoin; PoW is computer programming constituting the achievement (through both the generation and the transmission) of a relevant informational goal: to convey to all users the knowledge that Bitcoin is free of human tampering. Bitcoin's development community researches and develops Bitcoin protocol for some valuable practical goal. If there is no valuable practical goal, then there is a question as to why Bitcoin's community has worked on the PoW consensus algorithm for so many years. It is more reasonable, therefore, for one to commit to the claim that the programming of the PoW consensus algorithm was completed with a practical goal in mind. Additionally, since the PoW consensus algorithm is an information system technology, we have reason to claim it has the practical aim of achieving relevant information. The information goal is to inform everyone on the network that the Bitcoin ledger is free of human compromise.

The PoW consensus algorithm computer programming generates knowledge by directing a miner to find a solution—the nonce—to a cryptographic puzzle. During the miner's work, the PoW consensus algorithm measures the amount of computing power relative to a certain amount of time that it took for this miner to produce a block. This piece of information is then broadcast to the entire network, constituting the first form of transmission driven by the PoW algorithm. By competently generating and transmitting the solution to the cryptographic puzzle—the correct nonce —the other nodes in the network receive the solution. The nodes then add the new block to their respective ledger.

The PoW consensus algorithm ensures that each node needs to spend time and computational power to mine each block. This ensures that no one node can out-mine the most active Bitcoin ledger. The PoW computer programming ensures there is no overpowering node in the network by using the generated and transmitted information from each miner to calculate an overall metric; specifically, the PoW consensus algorithm evaluates how many blocks the network mined. Overall, then, the PoW consensus algorithm competently generates knowledge by coordinating all miners to send information about computing power spent mining blocks; furthermore, the PoW consensus algorithm competently transmits this knowledge to a calibration period every 2 weeks, whereby the difficulty level changes depending on whether the network mines blocks faster or slower than the standardized 2016 blocks/2 weeks. These steps are pieces of information that convey that the Bitcoin network is free from human tampering. This is because the POW consensus algorithm prevents any one entity from gaining power over the network, the POW consensus algorithm prevents human tampering, which is carried out through a computing power. In other words, if no computer can exert its power over the Bitcoin network, then no person can tamper with the Bitcoin ledger.

Since PoW's practical goal is to competently generate and transmit knowledge that Bitcoin's blockchain ledger is free from human tampering, when it accomplishes this goal, it can be seen as an "achievement." Knowledge generation and transmission, therefore, becomes an achievement that gives credit to the joint agency of all agents who contributed to the generation and transmission of that knowledge [41]. With regard to the PoW consensus algorithm, this achievement or credit can be seen in the way the Bitcoin cryptocurrency is distributed to all miners who successfully mine blocks. Recent evidence shows that in 2021 Bitcoin miners made upwards of $50 million a day mining blocks; furthermore, the total market cap value of Bitcoin reached over $ 1 trillion in 2021 [42].

One can evaluate a consensus algorithm's achievement by how competently the consensus algorithm's computer programming generates and transmits knowledge that its ledger is free of human tampering. This achievement is credit that goes to all agents who jointly operated the consensus algorithm's programming, generated blocks, and transmitted those blocks to all others. The immense value of Bitcoin and other blockchain cryptocurrencies is strong proof of the competence of their consensus algorithm. Cryptocurrency, therefore, represents this credit, which is to say the cryptocurrency's respective blockchain consensus algorithm. A blockchain protocol's native cryptocurrency, therefore, can represent the consensus algorithm's competence: the more cryptocurrency there is, the more epistemically competent the consensus algorithm is.

Another line of reasoning conveying the consensus algorithm's blockchain ledger is free of human tampering comes from the point of view of a wager. Bitcoin has had a market cap of over $1 trillion. This is more money that some countries have in their treasury and is more money than any one person in the world has. Malicious actors are motivated to do everything possible to try to tamper with Bitcoin's ledger in order to take even a small percentage of that $1 trillion. Yet since Bitcoin's launch in 2009, no human has successfully tampered with the Bitcoin ledger. If human tampering were at all possible, we have reason to believe it would already have happened. Since $1 trillion continues to be secure from any human tampering, it is reasonable to believe that an IOMT on-chain digital identity–which has far less monetary incentive for interference—will be secure from human tampering.

It is worth noting that the PoW consensus algorithm is competent at eliminating human tampering due to faulty human *ID Proofing*. An on-chain IOMT digital identity would eliminate the need for humans to carry out additional *ID Proofing* of the IOMT device after the manufacturer's ID Proofing at the point of manufacturing [43]. This means that the moment a manufacturer carries out an IOMT device's ID Proofing, this IOMT digital identity will retain its 1:1 correspondence with the respective IOMT device. Researchers testing a blockchain-based identity for products used in manufacturing and distribution found that 99.99% of the products retained their 1:1 correspondence with the correct product's digital identity, showing the competence of the blockchain consensus algorithm [22].

To sum up, competence in the generation and transmission of knowledge is attributed to an underlying process if and only if the underlying process generates and transmits knowledge that is relevant to the practical goals of the information economy. The PoW consensus algorithm, therefore, has a competent underlying computer programming that constitutes the competent generation and transmission of knowledge to users that Bitcoin's ledger is free of human tampering; this competence is represented by cryptocurrency and the precise accuracy of ensuring digital identities maintain a 1:1 correspondence to their underlying physical object. There has been no incident of PoW's consensus algorithm generating and transmitting knowledge that was not relevant to the practical aim of the Bitcoin network; specifically, the PoW consensus algorithm has allowed for the profitability of accruing Bitcoin's cryptocurrency. If this cryptocurrency is not compromised by human tampering, it seems fair to assume Bitcoin algorithm is a competent algorithm that reliability allows users to collect tokens of PoW's competent computer programming, generation, and transmission; furthermore, the competence of PoW supporting an information economy is a reliable process that supports the overarching justificatory mechanism of computational reliabilism. This is because it is more likely PoW's algorithmic competence protected Bitcoin from being stolen by securing the Bitcoin ledger from human tampering than it is that PoW accomplished this security by pure luck.

Measurement Robustness

Finally, computational reliabilism can be viewed through the lens of measurement theory. To contextualize such an approach, imagine asking ten different individuals what time it was based on the time indicated by their individual wristwatches. If eight of those ten individuals reported the same time, it would indicate a convergence of evidence, suggesting the watches were calibrated correctly. This is true regardless of whether or not the time indicated by this convergence is actually the time, since convergence is a calibration mechanism, not a tool for measuring reality. This convergence of evidence is what philosopher James Woodward calls measurement robustness [44]. This section, therefore, sees the PoW consensus algorithm as a measurement system that provides measurement robustness–suggesting a lack of human bias.

We begin by understanding the blockchain network as an "information machine." Metrologist Luca Mari argued in 1977 that information systems could be seen as measurement systems, giving precedent for our interpretation [45]. First, an input signal goes through a transformation to an output signal. In the case of Bitcoin, the information machine's operation occurs during the mining of the correct nonce. The input signal (the previous hash + the digital identity + the nonce to be discovered) is then converted by the hash function into a hash with the requisite number of difficulty zeroes. The PoW algorithm directs each miner to find the "right" input; in this case, the command to create a transformation that has an output with a hash of the previous block's hash and digital identity with the requisite number of difficulty zeroes. When the PoW directs each miner to use computational power to search (mine) for the right input, it also directs each miner to record the computational power used to find the right input.

PoW further refines what constitutes the "right" input at a macro level by aggregating the measurements from each miner and calculating the computational power it takes for the Bitcoin network to mine blocks in a two-week period. The measurand is the computational power used by each miner, while the measure is the amount of computational power used by each miner relative to a two-week time frame. This measure is established by a prescribed transformation; in the case of PoW, this prescribed transformation is 2016 blocks/2 weeks, which can be understood as PoW's calibration standard (one can view the calibration standard of 2016blocks/2 weeks as being similar to the standard of boiling water being 100C). 2016 blocks/2 weeks functions as an ideal result to compare experimental results. At two weeks, PoW compares the amount of blocks to the ideal number of blocks (thus 2016 blocks/2 weeks). Based on these results, PoW calibrates the network through difficulty.

It is important to note that 2016 blocks/2 weeks is what PoW uses to calibrate each miner. At the miner level, the prescribed transformation/1 miner is 1 block/10 min; that is, PoW prescribes each miner to transform an input into an output in 10 min. Thus, one can understand each miner as an independent PoW measurement instrument that calibrates itself to produce 1 block/10 min; consequently, each miner repeatedly affirms their measurements are free of human tampering through the principle of measurement robustness [44].

This being said, measurement robustness only works if there are enough miners that are independently controlled– that is, there are many people that operate the mining nodes, which are here treated as independent measurement instruments. Since miners are independent of each other, each node represents an independent measurement instrument. Every two weeks, the independent measurement instruments are calibrated in order to compute 1 block/10 min. Once the two-week interval begins, each node measures its own computational power. At the end of that two-week period, each node offers a measurement result of the actual time it took to compute blocks in two weeks relative to the ideal rate of 1 block/10 min. (This measurement of power output is the "work" that gives rise to the term proof of work). If the miners' measurement results have minimal fluctuations between them, then there is a convergence of evidence, indicating both that the convergent nodes were calibrated correctly and that there is minimal human bias. Our measurement results can be said to have measurement robustness, suggesting that the network has not been subject to human tampering.

PoW produces convergence of evidence of its own measurement calibration almost constantly since the mining nodes constantly mine—or, as described above, measure their own computing power. In turn, this generates a long history of convergence of evidence, indicating limited bias involved in the measurement process and providing pharmacovigilance decision makers with an additional reliable process. It is more likely that PoW directs the mining nodes—measurement instruments—to produce convergence of evidence due to the lack of human tampering, then it is that this convergence of evidence occurred due to pure luck.

Most importantly, PoW's measurement process is directly connected to the integrity of the IOMT digital identity. If the PoW measurement process is free from human tampering, then the IOMT digital identity itself is free from human tampering. We can draw this conclusion since the hash functions distribute the nonce, which is produced, in part, by the IOMT's digital identity. If one node tampers with the Bitcoin ledger and changes the IOMT's digital identity, then the measurement results will be different from all the other miner's measurement results: the node with a tampered digital identity will not produce results that offer measurement robustness. The PoW algorithm ensures that only the measurements that converge due to the cryptographically uniform ledger are admitted to the calibration that occurs every two weeks.

Conclusion

As we have shown, pharmacovigilance decision makers can justifiably rely on an on-chain IOMT digital identity being free from human tampering. The cryptographic science behind blockchain-based IOMT digital identities secures the digital provenance to the manufacturer's ID Proofing, ensuring that the digital identity is accurate and authentic. Furthermore, Proof of Work protects the digital identity from human tampering by ensuring it is computationally infeasible to change the cryptographically secure provenance of the digital identity. The PoW algorithm has unique epistemic implications that provide pharmacovigilance decision makers with a solution to a wicked problem; specifically, pharmacovigilance decision makers can leverage BCR to justify reliance through epistemic resources found within their system of beliefs. We have analyzed three such epistemic resources: appeal to expertise, algorithmic competence, and measurement robustness. Consequently, pharmacovigilance decision makers can overcome the wicked problem by using epistemic resources that they accept, thus providing them with standards of evaluating an emerging technology like blockchain based digital identities.

There is an important caveat, however, to ensuring a viable blockchain-based future for IOMT devices: choosing among the staggering array of blockchain-based protocols. While our essay has used Bitcoin Protocol as a focal point of analysis, there is, as we have mentioned, a great diversity of protocols in the blockchain industry. Each protocol is not the same; certain blockchain protocols are better suited for certain tasks. The cyber-physical realm is heterogeneous and complex in its technological process. This complexity and heterogeneity increase with the addition of all the blockchain protocols available. The task of justifying one blockchain protocol over another threatens to pose its own wicked problem for decision makers.

One of the most important considerations in choosing a blockchain-based protocol should be blockchain interoperability, a critical component for proper cybersecurity and physical convergence of all the industry 4.0 technologies, including the emerging pharmacovigilance 4.0 industry. By deploying technologies using interoperable blockchain protocols, pharmacovigilance decision makers can ensure their digital identity data does not get trapped in data siloes commonly seen in the United States Healthcare system [46, 47]. There is also a larger epistemic issue associated with blockchain protocols that are not interoperable. As seen in this essay, accuracy and authenticity are important for on-chain identities to have for decision making. If there is no blockchain interoperability, however, there is a risk that on-chain data will lack portability [48]. Therefore, by considering blockchain interoperability at the moment of considering blockchain technologies, pharmacovigilance can establish the right conditions for maximal usage of blockchain technology's epistemic value for decision making.

References

1. World Health Organization. Managing the COVID-19 infodemic: promoting healthy behaviours and mitigating the harm from misinformation and disinformation [Internet]. www.who.int. 2020 [cited 2021 Nov 4]. Available from: https://www.who.int/news/item/23-09-2020-managing-the-covid-19-infodemic-promoting-healthy-behaviours-and-mitigating-the-harm-from-misinformation-and-disinformation
2. WHO. Diagnostics laboratory emergency use listing [Internet]. www.who.int. 2021 [cited 2021 Nov 4]. Available from: https://www.who.int/teams/regulation-prequalification/regulation-and-safety/pharmacovigilance
3. Anne-Françoise Rutkowski (2018) Saunders CS. Emotional and Cognitive Overload: the Dark Side of Information Technology. Routledge, Abingdon, Oxon ; New York, NY
4. Bongomin O, Gilibrays Ocen G, Oyondi Nganyi E, Musinguzi A, Omara T (2020) exponential disruptive technologies and the required skills of industry 4.0. Dincer K, editor. J Eng 7:4280156
5. Goldman AI (2012) Reliabilism and contemporary epistemology: essays [Internet]. New York: Oxford University Press, 384 p. Available from: https://doi.org/10.1093/acprof:oso/9780199812875.001.0001/acprof-9780199812875
6. Becker K (2020) Reliabilism|internet encyclopedia of philosophy [Internet]. Internet encyclopedia of philosophy. [cited 2020 Mar 15]. Available from: https://iep.utm.edu/reliabil/
7. Durán JM (2018) Trusting computer simulations. Front Collection 79–111
8. Durán JM, Formanek N (2018) Grounds for trust: essential epistemic opacity and computational reliabilism. Mind Mach 28(4):645–666
9. Durán JM, Jongsma KR (2020) Who is afraid of black box algorithms? On the epistemological and ethical basis of trust in medical AI. J Med Ethics; medethics-2020-106820
10. Goldberg SC (2010) Relying on others: an essay in epistemology [Internet].Oxford University Press, Oxford, 240 p. Available from: https://doi.org/10.1093/acprof:oso/9780199593248.001.0001/acprof-9780199593248
11. Goldberg SC (2018) To the best of our knowledge: social expectations and epistemic normativity [Internet]. Oxford University Press, Oxford, 304 p. Available from: https://doi.org/10.1093/oso/9780198793670.001.0001/oso-9780198793670

12. Grassi PA, Garcia ME, Fenton JL (2017) Digital identity guidelines: revision 3. 2017 Jun 22; Available from: https://nvlpubs.nist.gov/nistpubs/SpecialPublications/NIST.SP.800-63-3.pdf
13. Eriksson O, Ågerfalk PJ (2021) Speaking things into existence: ontological foundations of identity representation and management. Inf Syst J 32(1):33–60
14. Kaur MJ, Mishra VP, Maheshwari P (2019) The convergence of digital twin, IoT, and machine learning: transforming data into action. Int Things 23:3–17
15. Cheung K-F, Bell MGH, Bhattacharjya J (2021) Cybersecurity in logistics and supply chain management: an overview and future research directions. Transp Res Part E: Logist Transp Rev 1(146):102217
16. Främling K, Harrison M, Brusey J, Petrow J (2007) Requirements on unique identifiers for managing product lifecycle information: comparison of alternative approaches. Int J Comput Integr Manuf 20(7):715–726
17. Sarkis M, Bernardi A, Shah N, Papathanasiou MM (2021) Emerging challenges and opportunities in pharmaceutical manufacturing and distribution. Processes 9(3):457
18. Srai JS, Kumar M, Graham G, Phillips W, Tooze J, Ford S et al (2016) Distributed manufacturing: scope, challenges and opportunities. Int J Prod Res 54(23):6917–6935
19. Islam MR, Aktheruzzaman KM (2020) An analysis of cybersecurity attacks against internet of things and security solutions. J Comput Commun 08(04):11–25
20. Das S, Siroky GP, Lee S, Mehta D, Suri R (2021) Cybersecurity: the need for data and patient safety with cardiac implantable electronic devices. Heart Rhythm 18(3):473–481
21. Klonoff D, Kerr D, Mulvaney SA (2020) Diabetes digital health. 1st ed. Elsevier, Amsterdam; Cambridge, Ma
22. Rao S, Gulley A, Russell M, Patton J (2021) On the quest for supply chain transparency through Blockchain: lessons learned from two serialized data projects. J Bus Logist
23. Michael WC (2021) Counterfeit drugs: a major issue for vulnerable citizens throughout the world and in the United States. J Am Pharm Assoc 61(1):e93–e98
24. Uddin M (2021) Blockchain Medledger: Hyperledger fabric enabled drug traceability system for counterfeit drugs in pharmaceutical industry. Int J Pharm 597:120235
25. Córdoba JSH, de J (2021) WSJ news exclusive | pfizer identifies fake Covid-19 shots abroad as criminals exploit vaccine demand. Wall Street Journal [Internet]. 2021 Apr 21 [cited 2021 Nov 4]; Available from: https://www.wsj.com/articles/pfizer-identifies-fake-covid-19-shots-abroad-as-criminals-exploit-vaccine-demand-11619006403
26. Erickson J (2008) Hacking: the art of exploitation, 2nd edn. No Starch Press, San Francisco, California
27. Collier ZA, Sarkis J (2021) The zero trust supply chain: managing supply chain risk in the absence of trust. Null 59(11):3430–45
28. Milkovich D (2020) 15 alarming cyber security facts and stats | cybint [Internet]. Cybint solutions - a BARBRI company. 2020 [cited 2021 Nov 4]. Available from: https://www.cybintsolutions.com/cyber-security-facts-stats/
29. Durán JM (2018) Computer simulations in science and engineering. Springer International Publishing, The Frontiers Collection. Cham
30. Ofori AY, Akoto D (2020) Digital forensics investigation jurisprudence: issues of admissibility of digital evidence. J Forensic Legal Invest Sci 6(1):1–8
31. Rietjens S (2022) Hybrid CoE a warning system for hybrid threats—is it possible? Hybrid CoE strategic analysis 22 [Internet]. 2020 [cited 2022 Apr 11]. Available from: https://www.hybridcoe.fi/wp-content/uploads/2020/06/Strategic-Analysis_22_WarningSystem-1.pdf
32. Furlonger D, Uzureau C (2019) The real business of blockchain : how leaders can create value in a new digital age. Harvard Business School Publishing Corporation, Boston
33. Franco P (2015) Understanding bitcoin: crytography, engineering and economics, 1st edn. Wiley, Chichester
34. Schneier B, Diffie W (2015) Applied cryptography: protocols, algorithms, and source code in C. Indianapolis (Ind.): Wiley, Cop
35. van Flymen D (2020) Learn blockchain by building one. Apress, Berkeley, CA

36. Kuhn TS (1996) The structure of scientific revolutions. 3rd ed. University of Chicago Press
37. Durán J (2014) Explaining simulated phenomena. A defense of the epistemic power of computer simulations
38. Parkin J (2020) Money code space: hidden power in bitcoin, blockchain, and decentralisation [Internet]. New York: Oxford University Press, 312 p. (OXFORD STUDIES DIGITAL POLITICS SERIES). Available from: https://doi.org/10.1093/oso/9780197515075.001.0001/oso-9780197515075
39. Leible S, Schlager S, Schubotz M, Gipp B (2019) A review on blockchain technology and blockchain projects fostering open science. frontiers in blockchain [Internet]. 2019 Nov 19;2. Available from: https://doi.org/10.3389/fbloc.2019.00016/full
40. Guo Y-M, Huang Z-L, Guo J, Guo X-R, Li H, Liu M-Y et al (2021) A bibliometric analysis and visualization of blockchain. Futur Gener Comput Syst 116:316–332
41. Greco J (2020) The Transmission of knowledge [Internet]. Cambridge University Press, Cambridge. Available from: https://www.cambridge.org/core/books/transmission-of-knowledge/FCF9A68D4B13E5127FD968CDE388FB0C
42. Chavez-Dreyfuss G, Wilson T (2021) Bitcoin hits $1 trillion market cap, surges to fresh all-time peak. Reuters.com. https://www.reuters.com/article/us-crypto-currency-bitcoin/bitcoin-hits-1-trillion-market-cap-surges-to-fresh-all-timepeak-idUSKBN2AJ0GC
43. Fernández-Caramés TM, Blanco-Novoa O, Froiz-Míguez I, Fraga-Lamas P (2019) Towards an autonomous industry 4.0 warehouse: a UAV and blockchain-based system for inventory and traceability applications in big data-driven supply chain management. Sensors 19 (10):2394
44. Woodward J (2006) Some varieties of robustness. J Econ Methodol 13(2):219–240
45. Mari L (1999) Notes towards a qualitative analysis of information in measurement results. Measurement 25(3):183–192
46. Dhaya R, Devi M, Kanthavel R, AlGarni F (2019) Big data analysis and management in healthcare. Data Sci 26:127–157
47. Birnbaum D (2019) Big data challenges from a public health informatics perspective. In: Househ M, Kushniruk AW, Borycki EM (eds) Big data, big challenges: a healthcare perspective: background, issues, solutions and research directions [Internet]. Springer International Publishing, Cham, pp 45–54. Available from https://doi.org/10.1007/978-3-030-06109-8_4
48. Belchior R, Vasconcelos A, Guerreiro S, Correia M (2021) a survey on blockchain interoperability: past, present, and future trends. ACM Comput Surv [Internet]. 54(8). Available fromhttps://doi.org/10.1145/3471140

Potential Implementations of Blockchain Technology in Patient Safety: A High-Level Overview

8

Minuette A. Laessig, Kushee-Nidhi Kumar, Wayne Bauerle, Stanislaw P. Stawicki, Shanaya Desai, Kimberly Costello, and Laurel Erickson-Parsons

An incident is just the tip of the iceberg, a sign of a much larger problem below the surface.

—Don Brown

Abstract

Blockchain technology (BCT), or more specifically its ability to maintain an immutable distributed ledger, is uniquely suited to a broad range of applications within patient safety. Potential use cases include, but are not limited to, medication safety, patient identification, event tracking, critical inventory management, internet-of-things (IoT), with many other potential uses to be explored. In this chapter, we explore key applications and considerations related to blockchain technology use in the area of patient safety. In addition to outlining potential existing and future use cases, we will also dedicate a

M. A. Laessig (✉)
Medical School of Temple University/St. Luke's University Health Network, Bethlehem, PA, USA
e-mail: tun07752@temple.edu

K.-N. Kumar · W. Bauerle · S. P. Stawicki · S. Desai
Department of Research and Innovation, St. Luke's University Health Network, Bethlehem, PA, USA

K. Costello · L. Erickson-Parsons
Department of Pediatrics, St. Luke's University Health Network, University Campus Bethlehem and Richard A. Anderson Campus, Easton, PA, USA

© The Author(s), under exclusive license to Springer Nature Switzerland AG 2023
S. Stawicki (ed.), *Blockchain in Healthcare*, Integrated Science 10,
https://doi.org/10.1007/978-3-031-14591-9_8

significant portion of the chapter to known and proposed implementations of blockchain technology across healthcare environments, both clinical and non-clinical.

Keywords

Blockchain technology · Innovation · Internet-of-Things · Patient safety

Introduction

Patient safety is a highly heterogeneous discipline spanning multiple domains within healthcare operations, form bedside care to medical transportation and various supply chains [1–4]. As in any highly complex system, communication (or lack thereof) tends to be among the chief contributing factors to failure [5, 6]. Critical information flows require meticulous cross-checking and sustained focus to achieve sustainable failure-free intervals. Within this context, the emergence of blockchain technology (BCT) provided the medical community with a new and highly powerful tool to help augment our ability to attain such sustained "zero defect" performance. In this chapter, we will discuss various existing and proposed applications of BCT in the area of patient safety, focusing on blockchain's ability to record immutable and highly accurate data in a distributed network of witness nodes, thus preventing the ability to tamper or otherwise influence any chain-of-evidence or critical information elements.

Brief Overview of Blockchain Technology

Blockchain technology (BCT) is based on the creation and maintenance of an immutable, anonymous, distributed ledger that additively stores data based on a pre-specified consensus mechanism to which independent nodes within the network subscribe [7–10]. None of the participating nodes controls the network, thus ensuring that only consensus-based operations can be performed. Consequently, any attempts at overriding, modifying, or otherwise altering data will be "detected and reverted" by the independent yet interconnected network participants.

Each blockchain transaction, stored in a so-called "block," has several key components: a hash, the hash of the previous block, a timestamp, and the data of the transaction(s) [11, 12]. The transaction data can be stored within the blockchain, or within an encrypted link [13, 14]. A hash is a fixed-length encryption output that represents the content of the block, commonly referred to as the block's "finger-print". Since each block includes the hash of the previous block (except for the special case of a "genesis block" or "block zero"), transactions are irreversible and linked together chronologically. If data in a block are changed it will generate a new hash and all subsequent blocks will be invalid—this is one security feature in blockchain that prevents tampering and double spending (in case of cryptocurrencies) [7, 15]. Blockchain can be viewed as a string of connected lights, each light is a block of transactions and the string that holds them together represents their link to every previous block via the hash. When one light on the string is damaged the subsequent lights will also go dark—signaling to everyone in the room that there is something wrong with the damaged light causing the rest in the string to go dark. Because it is decentralized and each "node" or "witness" contains its own copy of the entire chain, the affected node can be reconstituted based on information provided by all the other "witnesses" or "nodes" contributing their data toward that end. This also makes blockchain tamper-resistant (e.g., the presence of "witnesses" that share and auto-correct data results in the chain's ability to "defend" its integrity and internal consistency).

In addition to the blocks being linked together, proof-of-work (PoW) is added as an extra layer of security. Proof-of-work is a complex mathematical puzzle that introduces competition between network participants via competitive "mathematical puzzle solving" also known as "mining" [16, 17]. A majority of the nodes in the network have to "agree" on a block's validity before it is added to the chain. Mining activity is rewarded with "coins" (a.k.a., "unspent transaction outputs" or "UTXOs") and having a high amount of nodes mining the public ledger enhances the overall integrity of the system [18]. If previous blocks are tampered with, anyone who intends to alter the stored information (e.g., the hacker) would have to essentially "overpower and redo" the PoW for all following blocks and compete against the so-called "honest nodes" in the network. In effect, blockchains create a "trustless" network where information (e.g., transactions) are irreversible, anonymous, and practically immune to tampering [7–9, 15]. The PoW paradigm requires large amounts of energy and computing power, creating an environmental dilemma [19, 20]. Consequently, alternate methods of securing the blockchain have become much more popular, such as proof of stake (PoS), proof of participation (PoP) and proof of activity (PoA). Proof of participation uses a complex process to add nodes to the network and makes it more difficult for any malicious users to overtake the network while minimizing the computing power needed to uphold the peer-to-peer (P2P) network. Using proof of participation (PoP) in a private blockchain appears to be the most promising direction for EHR in healthcare since PoW requires set transactions per second and a large amount of computing power and energy [8, 13].

One core element of BCT is anonymity which is facilitated by the so-called "keys" (both public and private) that restrict access to information to a unique individual or key holder. Public keys are used to receive transactions and funds whereas private keys allow the end-user to spend funds (or send data) out of one's account [7]. In general, this broad area is called "public key cryptography" and is based on mathematical computations that are only solvable in "one direction," that is, public keys can be derived from private keys but the opposite is not possible (thus protecting one's identity, data and/or assets) [21, 22]. In a way, public keys are akin to one's post office box whereas private keys are required to open that post office box. What follows is that one would not be able to obtain access to the post office box solely by knowing its physical location. Much like in real life scenarios, if the physical key to open a post office box is not available, mail may continue to arrive but the addressee will not be able to retrieve it for personal use.

Blockchains can be public (e.g., permissionless), private (e.g., permissioned), hybrid (e.g., consortium) or sidechain (an offshoot of a "main" chain); Bitcoin is an example of a public blockchain where encrypted transactions are publicly visible [23, 24]. Private blockchains are typically controlled by a single organization and require permission from a system administrator to join the network and side chains allow asset transfer between blockchains [8, 14]. Private cloud-based data storage blockchains might be the future of medicine [22, 25], with a single administrator overseeing the blockchain and hospitals/trusted healthcare providers as the only "miners" or block validators, this model would decrease administrative costs and lead to more efficient operations [13].

Smart contracts are used within blockchain to irreversibly enforce pre-determined conditional agreements between parties. In healthcare, they can have a variety of applications such as recruiting patients for clinical trials, recording informed consent, designating patients at risk for falls, and flagging difficult airways [13, 26–29]. In healthcare, smart contracts could help facilitate performance-based reimbursements without cumbersome and inefficient communication patterns between healthcare workers and insurance companies [25]. In fact, Deloitte proposed a concept of BCT application in healthcare where institutions (e.g., hospitals, clinics) send patient information to the blockchain via Application Programming Interfaces (APIs) were patient information is stored and access is controlled by the patient, smart contracts are used to automatically pay for care, and researchers can use non-identifiable patient information for research [14].

Blockchain and Electronic Health Records

Currently deployed electronic medical record (EMR) systems are highly vulnerable and constantly face the risk of data breaches as well as internetwork incompatibility, leading to relative lack of patient trust and concerns over medical data safety [13, 30]. There has been an increase in health data breaches over the years, resulting mainly from hacking and unauthorized access incidents. Between 2009 and 2020 about 82% of United States citizens were victims of some form of health record breach. In 2020 alone there were 642 breaches resulting in exposure of > 500 individual records each [31]. These breaches may harm patient trust because in the current Health Information Exchange (HIE) system patients are unaware how information transfers occur [30], leading to ongoing concerns about losing control of personal data during HIE transactions/exchanges [32].

There are various systems designed to help track and protect patient information including electronic medical records (EMR), electronic health records (EHR), and personal health records (PHR) [33, 34]. Of those, EMR maintains internal records but does not foster communication between healthcare providers since the entirety of EMR data might not be transferred if the patient sees another provider [34]. Therefore, current systems make it difficult to piece together a complete patient history, impacting various aspects of patient care, including elements critical to patient safety such as reconciling information between healthcare providers and sharing of task- and diagnosis-critical data [25]. EHR systems generally foster better communication between various healthcare providers and thus tend to be less likely to contribute to medical errors [13, 35], although this is far from a universal rule. Moreover, current EHR systems may be more vulnerable when clinical information is being transferred between stakeholders. The most innovative form of health record today is the PHR, where patients furnish their own health data, either using automated tracking devices or some form of directed input [36]. This information is stored with their health history, enabling healthcare providers to use patient collected data to inform care. Because of some key properties common to both PHR and BCT (e.g., patient-controlled, highly secure, individualized), the PHR paradigm might be the future of blockchain technology implementations in patient health and preventative medicine [37, 38].

Blockchain technology may provide important solutions to some of the problems faced by the current EHR infrastructure. Blockchain technology was made popular by cryptocurrency and it is an immutable, anonymous, distributive ledger that records a chronological series of irreversible transactions [9]. Blockchain was popularized by Bitcoin, a cryptocurrency that uses a blockchain framework to secure transactions, however BCT has implications in a variety of areas such as entrepreneurship, voting, intellectual property [39], supply chain, energy sales, and healthcare [40, 41]. Blockchain in healthcare has the potential to connect providers, insurance companies, research organizations, and patients in a secure way that benefits all stakeholders [15, 25]. Though the public's knowledge of blockchain is commonly cited as a potential barrier [15], a recent study shows patients have a generally positive view of using BCT for their health information [30]. Blockchain technology offers solutions to challenges faced by EHRs via creating a trustless network with reduced transaction costs and smart contracts for consistent payment [7, 8, 25]. Blockchain also provides privacy and anonymity via cryptographic identification, all while fostering interoperability between networks [14]. In addition, BCT would be able to give physicians concise data about the patient, rather than the provider being overwhelmed by an overwhelming amount of data with limited relevance to the current episode of care [25]. Blockchain technology also poses an interesting solution for the secure long-term storage and distribution of health records.

Blockchain coupled with other related applications like smart contracts could help streamline healthcare payments; if a certain procedure is performed the program will automatically trigger billing for that procedure.

Surgical Applications of Blockchain

In surgery, blockchain technology has the possibility to streamline research, help predict surgical risk, promote safe anesthesia, and prevent common sentinel events such as retained surgical objects (RSIs) and wrong site surgery. A 2015 study found that 19% of clinical trials stopped because of failure to enroll, and that better systems for reaching patients could help this issue [42]. Blockchain with smart contracts is a feasible model of recruitment for clinical trials; with the blockchain system the patients just need to opt in for notifications of trials that could work for them and patients can consent with their private key [27]. Hopefully blockchain technology will connect more clinical trials to patients across all socioeconomic statuses, since this has been cited as an issue in clinical trials [43]. In addition, patients can easily consent to researchers adding their data without any protected health information or personal identifiers to a database, streaming data collection [14, 44]. With blockchain technology it is easier to access patients for consent, and patients tend to allow their data to be used for research when they stand to benefit [13].

Using blockchain technology for health records could also facilitate and streamline tools such as the American College of Surgeons National Quality Improvement Program Surgical Risk Calculator [44]. This risk assessment is performed preoperatively to determine risk of specific complications [45] which would be enhanced with blockchain-based health record, especially since blockchain would store an easily searchable complete medical history. When utilized optimally, these technologies could help patients and physicians alike to weigh the risks and benefits of surgery. Blockchain-based EHR implementations could make it much easier to examine medical records across a patient's life, inclusive of special medical and surgical precautions, such as the presence of difficult airway (for anesthesiologists) or previous metallic implant history (for magnetic resonance imaging) [29]. Smart contracts can be programmed into the blockchain such that, for example, patients with difficult airways or other complications are flagged to reduce systemic failures in anesthesia [46].

According to recent research approximately 20% of anesthesiologists report experiencing medication errors [47] and such errors are the leading cause of harm in healthcare [48]. In 2017, the World Health Organization (WHO) launched an initiative to reduce medication errors 50% over 5 years. Rather than blaming the individual, the WHO recognizes the importance of improving the systems, processes, and procedures to increase patient safety [48]. When medications are prescribed on patient floors, it typically goes through multiple steps (and through a chain of individuals) before administration, whereas in surgery the anesthesiologist completes multiple complex steps alone, often under significant stress and cognitive load [49]. Blockchain technology and machine learning can be used together to assist in anesthesia decision-making, which may help reduce the work for operating room teams and is intended to improve patient safety [50].

Sentinel events are patient safety events that results in death, permanent harm, or severe temporary harm [6, 51, 52], some of the most common surgical sentinel events in 2020 include retained surgical object (2nd most common event, 106 cases) and wrong site surgery (5th most common 68 cases) in the United States [53]. The highest number of wrong site surgeries occur in clinical areas that involve procedure-specific laterality, such as orthopedic surgery [54].

When sentinel events occur it is tempting to blame the event solely on an individual but this does not address systemic failures that may have contributed. This "Swiss cheese" model of failures states that failures occur when holes across different safety "levels" line up, specifically active failures (e.g., failures of healthcare professionals) and latent conditions (e.g., managerial, systemic, under-staffing) [55]. This "Swiss Cheese" model posits that a proactive system is one that generalizes isolated incidents and fixes latent conditions contributing to these incidents [52]. Checklists are one simple and revolutionary way to reduce adverse events in medicine, the modern surgical checklist originated in aviation [52, 56]. The checklist was introduced to aviation when both the airplanes air travel industry operations became so complex, and the consequences of even the slightest mistakes being potentially devastating, that a standard system based on strict adherence to established policies and procedures needed to be developed [4, 57–59]. In 2009 the World Health Organization (WHO) published the surgical checklist protocol which consists of a "sign in" process before anesthesia, a time out before the first incision, and a "sign out" after closure while the patient is still in the operating room [60]. Clinical data showed that incorporating elements of the WHO Surgical checklist into the EHR led to increased compliance and decreased risk events by 32% [61].

Recent studies showed that approximately 1 to 10 out of 10,000 surgeries are complicated by a retained surgical item (RSI) and systems such as sponge counting and surgical checklists may be effective in preventing RSIs [62, 63]. Blockchain technology can readily be incorporated into the overall safety verification process. For example, when both sponge counting and required checklists are completed, these important safety steps would be time stamped and stored in the blockchain, leading to both greater transparency and accountability. In addition, smart contracts using specialized HER interfaces and data abstraction could be used to flag cases for an increased risk of RSI. For example RSIs are more common in emergency surgery, multi-part procedures, surgery on a patient with a high BMI, and signifi-cant blood loss or other unexpected factors during surgery [64].

Wrong site surgery (WSS) is surgery involving either the incorrect anatomic part or incorrect patient is a truly disastrous surgical "never event" [65]. According to Hanchanale, "The surgeon should confirm the correct side with the clinic letter, consent form, theatre list, imaging studies, and also most importantly with the patient" [66]. In one study, out of 150 cases, sidedness was undocumented in clinic records for nearly 9% of cases and 5 records had the wrong side documented [66]. Though these errors did not necessarily lead to any WSS, easily accessing pertinent information and a full health history using blockchain-based EHR (or other dedi-cated safety systems) could optimally help flag any discrepancies and further pre-vent confusion and WSS. Blockchain could also be used to immutably document patient consent to the surgeries and surgical checklists adherence to encourage surgeons and surgical teams to follow the safety guidelines introduced by the WHO. Using specialized blockchain technology that interfaces with EHR has the potential to reduce latent errors in surgery by providing a more complete and highly transparent health history with clear time stamps to improve accountability for the required "sign in," "time out," and "sign out" safety huddles. Blockchain and smart contracts can also be used in a workflow system for documentation of pre-approvals, medical clearance, scheduling, preoperative testing and time-stamped consent [13, 28]. Using this technology would "simplify procedures, reduce administrative burdens and remove intermediaries" [41].

Blockchain in Medication Safety

With the utilization of separate EMRs at various institutions across the US, several logistical barriers to effective medical care emerged in the realm of medication prescribing and the associated medication safety. Common adverse medication events include incorrect drug dosing, the omission of a drug, and non-standard drug frequency, with nearly 8 out of 100 patients being affected by incorrect inpatient drug dispensing [67]. In the realm of outpatient care, medication non-adherence, controlled substance tracking, allergic reactions, and pharmacy reconciliation are critical barriers to providing safe and effective care to our patients [68, 69]. Currently, non-adherence rates are estimated to be in the range of 25%-50%, accounting for approximately $300 billion in healthcare-associated costs [68]. Non-adherence is a significant contributor to the progression of chronic conditions such as cardiovascular disease, chronic obstructive pulmonary disease, asthma, depression, diabetes, and human immunodeficiency virus, accounting for 125,000 deaths annually in the US alone [68, 70]. Blockchain technology provides an attractive and elegant solution to many of the previously mentioned issues. It was recently reported that a blockchain-based system designed specifically to track medication adherence is now available, providing a decentralized system for simple tracking [70]. Mitchell, et al., describe BMAR (blockchain medication administration records) use to help facilitate appropriate medication dispensing, medical observation, and audits whereas Li, et al., utilized a blockchain technology proof-of-concept to demonstrate a more accurate pharmacy reconciliation system compared to centralized systems [71, 72]. A decentralized BTC-based system has the potential to facilitate a more feasible, safe, and accurate pharmacologic treatment plan in several clinical settings such as inpatient, outpatient, as well as clinical trials. Even in its infancy, proof-of-concept blockchain models have demonstrated a more secure and cost-effective technology to enhance medication safety.

Prevention of Counterfeit Medications

Counterfeit medications are illegal, unsafe products that are fraudulently mislabeled and may contain incorrect or substandard ingredients [73]. It is estimated that 1%–2% of medications consumed world-wide are counterfeit and this illegal pharmaceutical production remains a lucrative business across the globe. Online pharmacies, unauthorized distribution channels, and limited inventory and stock visibility in the supply chain, amongst others, contribute to the challenges of ensuring product safety and controlling the industry. Blockchain technology has the potential to provide drug traceability for the stakeholders and track each transaction throughout the supply chain, ensuring accessibility, transparency and legitimacy of the end product [74, 75]. The decentralized distributed ledger creates a secure, time-stamped and immutable platform for direct digital transfers amongst the network of stakeholders across the pharmacy supply chain [76]. Significant investment, political backing, and stakeholder buy-in will need to be in place before effective BCT-based counterfeit medication prevention systems are in place.

Nuclear Medical Material Safety

The secure and decentralized method of storing data through blockchain technologies can prove itself to be very useful with nuclear material safety in nuclear medicine [77]. Much has been learned from past misadventures involving poor oversight and inadequate supply chain tracking involving medical nuclear isotopes [78]. Though nuclear medicine has a diagnostic and therapeutic capacity, appropriate vigilance must be maintained regarding potential misuse. Even and after significantly enhancing the overall safety and supply chain efficiency in this important area, nuclear materials must always be treated as hazardous materials that have the potential to cause undue radiation hazards to the public. This causes the handling, oversight, and transportation of nuclear materials to be a very critical task that involves not only patient safety but also the well-being of medical staff and the general public [77].

Using BCT can be potentially beneficial to tracking nuclear medical materials since each block of data can store important information with a timestamp that cannot be edited [79]. This, BCT can increase efficiency, trust, and transparency in the management of nuclear medicine supply chains [80]. With BCT, it may be possible to track the exact pathways of nuclear materials and ensure that they are being transferred in the safest and most efficient way possible [81]. Additionally, since blockchain has decentralized data storage, it makes it much more difficult for the nuclear material information to be compromised by malignant third-party actors [80].

Curtailing Drug Abuse with the Help of Blockchain

The United States, and many other parts of the world, are facing an acute opioid and drug abuse crisis [82, 83]. The costs, both human and economic, of this true epidemic, are truly staggering [84–86]. Development of suitable databases that provide secure, real-time access to key stakeholders dealing with the opioid crisis will be essential if the containment efforts are to be successful [87]. Blockchain technologies, with their inherent features of decentralization, immutability, and easy access are well suited to achieving these goals. Consequently, BCT-based solutions would help optimize critical communication and data aggregation between various EHRs, many of which not being inherently compatible. Some practical applications of blockchain technologies include data collection/aggregation/analysis, patient/provider identification, traceability/monitoring of opioids, supply chain provenance, prescription monitoring, licensure and credentialing, interoperability, seamless integration/communication, development of opioid alternatives, and research incentivization [83].

Blockchain-Based Patient Tracking

Not infrequently, patients with similar names or diagnoses undergo diagnostic testing and invasive procedures within a relatively small temporal space, creating the potential for a wrong-patient/wrong-test mismatch. On more than one occasion, similarly named patients undergo diagnostic tests, procedures, or admissions meant for another patient. The multiple layers of similarity between two patients and their clinical management may create the potential for mismatching patient information [88–92].

Some additional common overlaps between two similarly named patients include the time frame of admission and the proximity of their hospital room. For example, when two similarly named patients are in the same intensive care unit, their chance of being misidentified increases, therefore increasing the likelihood that a test or procedure is performed on the wrong individual. A qualitative analysis of the Veterans Health Administration reported that 182 out of 253 medical errors in a single cycle were due to patient misidentification. In that study, the most common misidentification errors included specimen mislabeling, misinformation during manual entry of the patients' data, and two-step verification failure [93]. Blockchain can help us overcome many of these barriers while at the same time reducing the amount of work and cognitive load required by our already busy healthcare teams. Moreover, a two-step verification system could be transitioned into a single/one identity verification system. Security and accuracy are ensured through a unique single identifier that is controlled by the patient or the staff that has access to the protected information [94, 95]. With a blockchain system in place, the amount of time spent verifying patient information decreases, and the number of errors entered in the system also inherently decreases. In essence, a BCT-based system could prevent the mismatching of patient tests, procedures, or specimens, and ultimately improving patient outcomes.

Visitor Tracking in Highly Sensitive Areas

Highly restricted areas, such as the operating suites, labor and delivery, intensive care units (from neonatal to adult settings) could easily incorporate BTC-based solutions to more effectively track the onboarding, tracking, and offboarding of visitors, with largely automated procedures that are much less likely to result in a security breach. Having a reliable security system in highly restricted hospital areas is critical to providing excellent quality of care. Blockchain-based prototypes using smart cards or other digital devices have been proposed as solutions to better control entry to restricted areas [96]. Additionally, Blockchain technology could be used in combination with biometrical data to allow trusted and secured access to individuals to highly restricted hospital areas [97].

For highly efficient and privacy-centric tracking systems, any required biometric data could be securely stored on a customized blockchain-based security device that permits only the holder to provide sensitive data. Such approach could allow family members to visit their loved ones while simultaneously reducing the concern for possible security and/or privacy breaches. Overall, blockchain could transform how healthcare facilities approach security for patient visitor tracking by creating unique identifiers to track the onboarding and off-boarding of visitors [98, 99].

Multiple Casualty Scenarios

When it comes to multi-casualty incidents (MCI) there exists a constant risk of patient identity mismatch, potentially leading to unacceptable clinical outcomes including delay-to-treatment, mistriage, long-term disability, and even loss-of-life [100, 101]. Easy-to-deploy tagging and workflow tracking systems built using existing BCT capacity are well-positioned to reduce the chaos and improve information flows during MCIs. Such systems could be based on barcode tagging, mobile devices, and would easily integrate into established electronic medical record systems. In terms of their fundamental functioning, such implementations would essentially utilize the internet-of-things (IoT) paradigm, with multiple simultaneously communicating devices and micro-devices within the MCI-affected area [102, 103]. Although it is understood broadly that patient safety might not be the top priority in a situation where multiple injured individuals are being cared for by an overwhelmed disaster response team, it must be emphasized that any tool that reduces the overall chaos and improves information flows during MCIs will inherently improve patient safety and quality of the emergency services provided.

Follow-Up and Long-Term Care

Blockchain technology provides a unique, platform-agnostic bridge to help consolidate and streamline long-term and follow-up care, especially across geographically remote settings (e.g., a traveler seen at one location but following-up elsewhere) and/or incompatible EMR systems (e.g., a patient seen by two different institutions, each using a different EMR) [104, 105]. Because blockchain can store highly secure, encrypted information using universal data storage formats, the public could benefit from the ability to safely and reliably share their medical records across different platforms, with the patient being firmly in control of their own medical information [106, 107]. Similar benefits translate into long-term care that potentially spans different settings and/or providers.

Real-Time Information Sharing Within the Internet-Of-Things (IoT) Paradigm

As outlined earlier in the current chapter, multiple interconnected devices working together—either within a specific geographic area or toward a specific purpose—can form a hive-like functionality that effectively functions as a supercomputer [108]. This mode of multi-device operations is also called "internet-of-things" or IoT [109]. Within such paradigm, various devices could feed data directly into a "data hive," which in turn could inform powerful computational algorithms that help guide physicians to improve both the quality and safety of bedside care.

The realm of possibilities within each IoT "microverse" is truly unlimited, and BCT provides an excellent platform for all the interconnected devices to become truly interoperative [110, 111]. A realistic outcome of an IoT implementation for patient safety may mean that real-time feedback from multiple inputs (e.g., various monitoring devices) is combined with real-time input from clinical bedside personnel (e.g., nursing observations) and transmitted instantaneously to an "alert/notification" system that identifies patient deterioration and the responsible physician. Of course, this is just a simple example of a fairly straight-forward system. Such paradigms could then be expanded into healthcare facility logistics (e.g., notification of need for critical a care bed; automated restocking of critical supplies; or even medical transportation scheduling and coordination across a region, etc.).

Immunity Certificates/passports

As shown repeatedly during the coronavirus disease 2019 (COVID-19) pandemic, the issues of vaccination and viral immunity can be very contentious [112–114]. Regardless of personal beliefs, the preponderance of scientific evidence points to the effectiveness and clear overall benefits of appropriate vaccination [115, 116]. That said, important challenges exist regarding one's ability to reliably produce (and permanently store) information that provides "proof of vaccination" or—for those who recovered from an infectious disease—"proof of immunity" [117].

Given that the current public health paradigm is evolving toward a universal vaccination requirement, it will be important to reliably, inexpensively, and easily prove one's "immunization status." There have also been proposals to entirely automate the process, whereby IoT-based systems using a variety of stationary and mobile devices could help track and "clear" one's "immunization status" without creating disruptions in various processes and/or workflows that would otherwise require interruption. Given the above, BCT is uniquely suited to provide such a solution, complete with full control of personal data resting with the information holder (e.g., the "immunity certificate" bearer) [117]. As such, blockchain-based implementations would both serve their intended function while protecting the holder's rights to privacy and self-determination.

Device Tracking/Identification

Combined with the above-mentioned IoT construct, BCT is well-suited for allowing medical devices to store privileged information with the assurance that the information remains secure. Details of product design and development/production may be stored and accessed by only those necessary. Blockchain-based technology also allows for better oversight of both the distribution and redistribution of devices to be traced—something that is important when devices are highly specialized and their misuse could prove dangerous to patients [118–120].

The practicality of this technology, including various security implications, far exceeds the concept of "a device." This is primarily because IoT-based "device networks" in healthcare applications will contain both sensitive patient and end-user data, including detailed logs of who used the device, why it was used, and when it was used [121, 122]. Aggregate data from various wearables, stationary monitors, and other sources, can then be used for a variety of purposes, including analysis of patient compliance, verification of healthcare provider notification and/or subsequent action, and finally multi-parametric device performance metrics and diagnostics [123–125]. This paradigm can be employed with both implantable medical devices and external medical devices. Examples of devices that contain individual patient data and may be able to benefit from blockchain technology are insulin pumps and continuous glucose monitors or glucometers that have the ability to store and track highly specific patient information including glucose levels and insulin usage [126, 127]. Medical images are another type of patient data that can be stored directly within medical equipment "memory" while at the same time fully leveraging the secure decentralized system of BCT by allowing authorized stakeholders to access pertinent images while at the same time keeping other patient information restricted [128]. Blockchain technology will make devices resistant to tampering and/or hacking thereby securing product and patient sensitive information. Institutions may also take advantage of using BCT to record mission-critical information such as instructions and safety information, including product recalls, safety protocols and procedures, and other related items. Such information can then be readily disseminated to all authorized users, without the need for any specialized infrastructure (other than simple Internet or Intranet access, as applicable/required).

Tracking of Product Expiration Dates

Patient safety is inherently tied to proper medical product handling, storage, usage, and lifecycle restrictions [129–131]. Currently, tracking expiration dates and/or potential harmful interactions for drugs and medical equipment is cumbersome and time consuming, with multiple opportunities for improvement [132, 133]. Blockchain technology potentially provides "the next step" in developing a more efficacious process that will drastically reduce the time and resources spent tracking expiration dates and product safety/viability. In the context of the current coronavirus disease 2019 (COVID-19) pandemic, vaccines are a particularly important area that accurate records of expiration dates and administration is essential for public health [134]. Modern messenger RNA (mRNA) vaccines are especially vulnerable to various supply chain interruptions [135]. The ability to securely store critical data, such as expiration dates, in a decentralized system that is both very secure and readily accessible, while restricting more sensitive product information, can be paradigm-changing compared to the current *status quo*. Moreover, the ability to scan the device, drug, or vaccine for access to the required information, provides multiple (and appropriately redundant) ways of tracking expiration dates (and other key safety parameters) while employing BCT.

Secure Transactions and Fraud Prevention

Initially implemented in the realm of "cryptocurrencies," blockchain is uniquely suited to provide robust capabilities in the areas of secure transactions and fraud prevention. Inherent to their immutability, BCT-based "transaction ledgers" are designed specifically to record and reproduce "proof" of any recordable transaction, whether that is "an event," "an acknowledgment," or "a document submission."

Consequently, blockchain-based platforms are uniquely positioned to help facilitate low-cost, secure transactions while at the same time reduce or eliminate fraud within the healthcare system. In addition, the blockchain's high specificity toward a specific object, individual, and/or transaction, all make it a very effective tool against unauthorized or erroneous transactions. Systemic implications for our healthcare facilities are significant, with various efficiencies enabling cost savings and more optimal reinvestment of scarce resources.

Blockchain Security and Patient Autonomy

Under the current paradigm of various forms of EMRs, patients are not able to fully own their health information and thus do not control the secure transfer of said information between healthcare professionals and/or facilities [10]. Privacy-optimized implementations of BCT could offer patients the ability to control own their own data and any access to such data via the control of one's individual "private keys" [136, 137]. Because the patient fully controls their medical information at all times, he or she can also revoke access at any time, thus giving more agency to the patient [13, 15, 30]. In one proposal, Deloitte advocates a software-based solution that provides the patient with the above-outlined powers. The same team also proposed that in emergency situations there would be prior authorizations in place so the healthcare team can access the entirety of the patient's data (a contingency restricted to situations when the patient is incapacitated) [14, 44]. Of increasing concern is the growing presence of malignant actors (e.g., hackers) who continue to develop highly creative ways to compromise confidential patient information. In cases of centralized EMR hacking, all patient records within that particular EMR system would be compromised; however, in a BCT-based system, hackers would be forced to attack individual patient records "one-by-one" [14], making the overall effort impractical, if not prohibitive in terms of time and resources needed to carry out a successful "attack." Moreover, evolving solutions such as Practical Swarm Optimization (PSO) featuring logitboost appear promising to identify private key hackers and further secure the blockchain [138, 139].

Estonia: An Example of Blockchain Implementation in Healthcare

Estonia is a small Baltic country that is home to approximately 1.3 million citizens [140]. The country is world renowned for being technologically advanced and is among the first to transition to BCT on a national level—a move prompted by cyberattacks in 2007 [141]. In the 1990's, healthcare providers started creating EHR systems but the various systems were unable to effectively exchange patient information—something that is all-too-familiar to the issues facing The United States and other developed country medical systems today. The Estonian government set out on a 4-point mission to address the issue: [a] creating electronic health records; [b] digital images; [c] digital registration; and [d] digital prescriptions. It has been reported that the newly implemented system improved both healthcare efficiency and patient safety, with estimated 15–17% of prescription-related drug interactions being prevented by specialized support software [142]. Today Estonia uses Keyless Signature Infrastructure (KSI) blockchain. The KSI approach uses the Unix philosophy of "abstraction and encapsulation of functionality into layers, each of which does one thing well" [143]. In turn, this provides a readily scalable technology that is capable of processing millions of transactions per second.

According to Estonia's government website the KSI technology allows 10^{12} items of data to be processed every second and relies on cryptographic proof rather than third party trust [7, 141]. Patients can access and share all of their health records on patient portals using their electronic ID cards, empowering the patient to be in control of their own health data.

Estonia is among the most technologically advanced healthcare systems in the world, yet still faces many systemic issues that need to be addressed, including access to healthcare and some degree of inefficiency [140]. While implementing the KSI blockchain EHR, Estonia faced a few roadblocks-such as system compatibility issues and some degree of staff apprehension. The system was implemented in 2008, and despite a relatively successful implementation process there were still some persistent "transition-related issues" as late as 2012 [140]. These seem to have been overcome, and the latest data from Estonia shows that 100% of billing is done electronically and 99% of health data is digitized [144]. Through their use of novel KSI blockchain technology to digitize health records, Estonia serves as small-scale, whole-country proof that blockchain can be successfully applied in healthcare [37].

Implementation Basics

Deloitte suggests a 4 part implementation framework for organizations interested in blockchain. These phases are as follows: [a] initiate (establish pre-conditions); [b] design (determine applications); [c] strengthen (use of smart contracts); and [d] implement (permissionless, permissioned, or consortium blockchains) [14]. In addition to this basic implementation framework, the authors of the repor suggest that consortiums should be created to invest in developing blockchain and to support any ongoing experimentation [14]. As mentioned previously, private blockchains using proof-of-participation (PoP) might be the most compatible with, and well-suited for, healthcare applications. There are various vendors developing blockchain healthcare solutions such as Doc.ai (Palo Alto, California); Encryptogen [15]; Logware (Charlotte, North Carolina); and Medicalchain (London, UK) [25]. For blockchain to be used widely and be easily accessible by multiple stakeholders, middleware should be in place to create a patient-friendly portal so patients can easily manage their own information [44]. It is recommended that incentives are provided for "nodes" (i.e., participants or stakeholders within the network) to invest computing power in the network and the computing power should be "as distributed as possible" to avoid any one node from monopolizing and/or subverting the network [44].

Important Limitations

Blockchain technology continues to face significant issues on its quest to achieve widespread adoption. These challenges include, but are not limited to, scalability, cost, regulation, upgradeability, addition and linking of new and existing data, and privacy [14, 145]. For a blockchain EHR to be widely adopted it needs to be scalable. This means that it would need sufficient computing power to handle millions of transactions per second, all whilst interfacing seamlessly with other healthcare information systems. Although private blockchains and KSI technology may allow more transactions per second, questions remain regarding the network's transactional throughput capacity given the healthcare's truly widespread (and continuously expanding) data processing needs. Interfacing with other healthcare systems is also not a trivial issue, and it is one that will likely take a great deal of technological support and innovation. In addition, transferring patient data from paper records and from existing EMRs to the blockchain would also involve a significant cost, time and effort.

Cost is also a significant potential limitation to BCT adoption in healthcare. Although blockchain would cut down on administrative costs by removing various inefficient intermediaries, current BCT such as Bitcoin takes more electricity to run than a small country [8]. In addition, extensive IT support and employee training would likely be needed to ensure that any implementation happens smoothly. For these reasons, the cost effectiveness of transitioning to a blockchain EHR continues to be debated [26]. New ways to secure the network such as PoP rather than PoW might result in a more efficient system that consumes less energy and overall computing power, which is certainly a very promising way forward. Nonetheless, the cost(s) of implementation, energy, and computing power are still valid concerns.

Blockchain still exists in a grey area of the law, making regulation and implementation somewhat difficult [145]. In addition, privacy is paramount to using blockchain in healthcare. In theory, BCT-based healthcare record implementation would mean that patients are the only ones that know their private keys, which keeps their data secure but also in itself restricts access. However if a patient loses their private key, they would also lose access to their healthcare data. One solution to this dilemma might be through creative implementations of a multisignature system, with a universal key kept by a trusted entity that could authorize occasional one-time retrieval of the patient's data into a new, "restored" blockchain record, but only upon the patient proving their identity to the entity, or when life-threatening emergency requires immediate access for life-saving interventions. In other words, without a recovery system patient data could be lost forever if the private key is not known, but at the same time some degree of privacy and confidentiality may need to be compromised to guarantee that "no harm" results from unintentional private key loss.

Conclusions

Blockchain technology represents an important step in human technological advancement. It is an immutable, anonymous, and secure way to complete transactions [9], with "any data or process" that is "measurable" and "recordable" being suitable for inclusion. Applying this technology to healthcare would allow patients to own their personal data and control who can access it [13, 15]. In this way blockchain would promote transparency between healthcare providers and patients. In addition, patients would have more complete healthcare records, without the discontinuous/partial records that plague the healthcare industry today. Having a complete health history is critical because reconciling information over multiple providers to "piece together" a patient history is costly, time consuming, often inaccurate, and prone to security breaches [25]. Estonia's success in implementing blockchain into healthcare is inspirational and they could serve as a small scale model for the other healthcare systems [37]. Although large-scale implementations of BCT in healthcare will likely prove difficult, this task is certainly not insurmountable. To successfully transition into the "healthcare mainstream," BCT-based systems will need to address concerns around scalability, cost, emergency access to data, regulation and privacy before they are widely used.

References

1. Panesar S et al (2014) Patient safety and healthcare improvement at a glance. Wiley
2. Buyurgan N, Farrokhvar P (2015) Supply chain-related adverse events and patient safety in healthcare. Int J Healthcare Inform Syst Informat (IJHISI) 10(2):14–33
3. Mattox E (2012) Medical devices and patient safety. Crit Care Nurse 32(4):60
4. Hon HH et al (2016) Injury and fatality risks in aeromedical transport: focus on prevention. J Surg Res 204(2):297–303
5. Stawicki SP et al (2014) Natural history of retained surgical items supports the need for team training, early recognition, and prompt retrieval. Amer J Surg 208(1):65–72
6. Stawicki SP et al (2019) Introductory Chapter: patient safety is the cornerstone of modern healthcare delivery systems. Vignettes Patient Safety 4:1–11
7. Crosby M, Pattanayak P, Kalyanaraman V (2016) Bitcoin technology: beyond bitcoin. Appl Innov Rev (2)
8. Darlington N (2021) Blockchain for beginners: what is blockchain technology? a step-by-step guide. Available from: https://blockgeeks.com/guides/what-is-blockchain-technology/
9. Nakamoto S (2008) Bitcoin: a peer-to-peer electronic cash system
10. Chen HS et al (2019) Blockchain in healthcare: a patient-centered model. Biomed J Sci Tech Res 20(3):15017–15022
11. Fill H-G, Härer F (2018) Knowledge blockchains: applying blockchain technologies to enterprise modeling. In: Proceedings of the 51st Hawaii international conference on system sciences
12. Aste T, Tasca P, Di Matteo T (2017) Blockchain technologies: the foreseeable impact on society and industry. Computer 50(9):18–28
13. Vazirani AA et al (2019) Implementing blockchains for efficient health care: systematic review. J Med Internet Res 21(2):e12439

14. Krawiec R et al (2016) Blockchain: opportunities for health care. Available from: file:///C:/Users/minla/Downloads/us-blockchain-opportunities-for-health-care.pdf.
15. Hughes A et al (2019) Beyond Bitcoin: what blockchain and distributed ledger technologies mean for firms. Bus Horiz 62(3):273–281
16. Huber T, Sornette D (2020) Boom, bust, and bitcoin: bitcoin-bubbles as innovation accelerators. Swiss Finan Inst Res Paper (20–41)
17. Warmke C (2021) What is bitcoin? Inquiry, 1–43
18. Tschorsch F, Scheuermann B (2016) Bitcoin and beyond: a technical survey on decentralized digital currencies. IEEE Commun Surv Tutorials 18(3):2084–2123
19. Vaughn R, Talukder S (2020) A template for useful proof of work. J Comput Sci Coll 36 (3):191–191
20. Bahri L, Girdzijauskas S (2018) When trust saves energy: a reference framework for proof of trust (PoT) blockchains. In: Companion proceedings of the the the web conference 2018
21. What Are Public and Private Keys? (2021). Available from: https://www.gemini.com/cryptopedia/public-private-keys-cryptography
22. Xia Q et al (2017) BBDS: blockchain-based data sharing for electronic medical records in cloud environments. Information 8(2):44
23. Bheemaiah K (2017) Fragmentation of finance. The Blockchain Alternative. Springer, pp 25–82
24. Krishnan S et al (2020) Handbook of research on blockchain technology. Academic Press
25. Sharma L et al (2021) How blockchain will transform the healthcare ecosystem. Bus Horizons
26. Giordanengo A (2019) Possible usages of smart contracts (Blockchain) in healthcare and why no one is using them. Stud Health Technol Inform 264:596–600
27. Zhuang Y et al (2019) Applying blockchain technology to enhance clinical trial recruitment. AMIA Annu Symp Proc 2019:1276–1285
28. Asma K (2020) A blockchain-based smart contract system for healthcare management. Electronics 9:94
29. Mandel J (2018) Engineering challenge. Soc Technol Anesthesia
30. Esmaeilzadeh P, Mirzaei T (2019) The potential of blockchain technology for health information exchange: experimental study from patients' perspectives. J Med Internet Res 21 (6):e14184
31. Healthcare Data Breach Statistics. [cited 2021; Available from: https://www.hipaajournal.com/healthcare-data-breach-statistics/
32. Kim KK, Joseph JG, Ohno-Machado L (2015) Comparison of consumers' views on electronic data sharing for healthcare and research. J Am Med Inform Assoc 22(4):821–830
33. Cahill JE, Gilbert MR, Armstrong TS (2014) Personal health records as portal to the electronic medical record. J Neurooncol 117(1):1–6
34. Heart T, Ben-Assuli O, Shabtai I (2017) A review of PHR, EMR and EHR integration: a more personalized healthcare and public health policy. Health Policy Technol 6(1):20–25
35. Han JE et al (2016) Effect of electronic health record implementation in critical care on survival and medication errors. Am J Med Sci 351(6):576–581
36. Roehrs A, da Costa CA, da Rosa Righi R (2017) OmniPHR: a distributed architecture model to integrate personal health records. J Biomed Inform 71:70–81
37. Williams-Grut O (2016) Estonia is using the technology behind bitcoin to secure 1 million health records. Available from: http://www.businessinsider.com/guardtime-estonian-health-records-industrial-blockchain-bitcoin-2016-3?r=UK&IR=T
38. Ichikawa D, Kashiyama M, Ueno T (2017) Tamper-resistant mobile health using blockchain technology. JMIR Mhealth Uhealth 5(7):e111
39. Stawicki S, Firstenberg M, Papadimos T (2018) What's new in academic medicine? Blockchain technology in health-care: Bigger, better, fairer, faster, and leaner. Int J Acad Med 4(1):1–11

40. Dutta P et al (2020) Blockchain technology in supply chain operations: applications, challenges and research opportunities. Transp Res Part E: Logist Transp Rev 142:102067
41. Khatoon A (2020) A blockchain-based smart contract system for healthcare management. Electronics 9(1):94
42. Carlisle B et al (2015) Unsuccessful trial accrual and human subjects protections: an empirical analysis of recently closed trials. Clin Trials 12(1):77–83
43. Sharrocks K et al (2014) The impact of socioeconomic status on access to cancer clinical trials. Br J Cancer 111(9):1684–1687
44. Peters A et al (2017) Blockchain technology in health care: a primer for surgeons. Bullet Amer College of Surgeons 102(12)
45. Surgical Risk Calculator. 2020 [cited 2021]; Available from: https://riskcalculator.facs.org/RiskCalculator/
46. Singh J, An N, Scher C (2018) ASACoin: a model cryptocurrency to highlight potential applications of blockchain technology to enhance outcomes in anesthesia delivery. Available from: http://www.asaabstracts.com/strands/asaabstracts/abstract.htm?year=2018&index=8&absnum=4762
47. Bratch R, Pandit JJ (2021) An integrative review of method types used in the study of medication error during anaesthesia: implications for estimating incidence. British J Anaesthesia
48. Medication without harm—global patient safety challenge on medication safety. 2017; Available from: https://apps.who.int/iris/bitstream/handle/10665/255263/WHO-HIS-SDS-2017.6-eng.pdf
49. Evley R et al (2010) Confirming the drugs administered during anaesthesia: a feasibility study in the pilot National Health Service sites. UK. Br J Anaesth 105(3):289–296
50. Yu Z, Liu Y, Zhu C (2021) Application of propofol in oral and maxillofacial surgery anesthesia based on smart medical blockchain technology. J Healthcare Eng 2021:11
51. Chen TC, Schein OD, Miller JW (2015) Sentinel events, serious reportable events, and root cause analysis. JAMA Ophthalmol 133(6):631–632
52. Stawicki S (2015) Fundamentals of patient safety in medicine and surgery. Wolters kluwer india Pvt Ltd
53. Sentinel event statistics released for 2020 (2021); Available from: https://www.jointcommission.org/resources/news-and-multimedia/newsletters/newsletters/joint-commission-online/march-24-2021/sentinel-event-statistics-released-for-2020/
54. Robinson PM, Muir LT (2009) Wrong-site surgery in orthopaedics. J Bone Joint Surg Br 91 (10):1274–1280
55. Reason J (2000) Human error: models and management. BMJ 320(7237):768–770
56. Smith E et al (2015) Surgical safety checklist: Productive, nondisruptive, and the " right thing to do". J Postgrad Med 61(3):214
57. Gawande A (2007) The checklist: if something so simple can transform intensive care, what else can it do? New Yorker, 86–101
58. Stawicki S, Hoey BA, Portner M (2013) Evidence tables: summary of aeromedical incidents (2003–2012). OPUS 12:3–15
59. Anagnostakos JP et al (2014) Evidence tables: Summary of aeromedical incidents (2013–2014). OPUS 8:9–16
60. WHO Surgical Safety Checklist (2009) World Health Organization
61. Using the WHO Surgical Safety Checklist (2016); Available from: https://www.cardinalhealth.com/content/dam/corp/web/documents/case-study/cardinal-health–using-the-who-surgical-safety-checklist–5CR16-542008_2.pdf
62. Szymocha M et al (2019) Leaving a foreign object in the body of a patient during abdominal surgery: still a current problem. Pol Przegl Chir 91(6):35–40
63. Stawicki SP et al (2013) Retained surgical items: a problem yet to be solved. J Am Coll Surg 216(1):15–22

64. Moffatt-Bruce SD et al (2014) Risk factors for retained surgical items: a meta-analysis and proposed risk stratification system. J Surg Res 190(2):429–436
65. Lin A et al (2018) Wrong-site procedures: Preventable never events that continue to happen. Vignettes Patient Safety 2:2113
66. Hanchanale V et al (2014) Wrong site surgery! How can we stop it? Urol Ann 6(1):57–62
67. Rothschild JM et al (2010) Medication errors recovered by emergency department pharmacists. Ann Emerg Med 55(6):513–521
68. Iuga AO, McGuire MJ (2014) Adherence and health care costs. Risk Manag Healthc Policy 7:35–44
69. Hammad EA et al (2017) Pharmacy led medicine reconciliation at hospital: a systematic review of effects and costs. Res Social Adm Pharm 13(2):300–312
70. Madhusudan Singh D-KK, Lee J-H, Tiwary US, Singh D, Chung W-Y (2020) Intelligent human computer interaction, Vol 2. 2020: Springer
71. Hamid Jahankhani SK, Jamal A, Epiphaniou G, Al-Khateeb H (2019) Blockchain and clinical trial: securing patient data. Springer
72. Li P et al (2019) DMMS: a decentralized blockchain ledger for the management of medication histories. Blockchain Healthc Today 2
73. Sekhar MS et al (2011) Counterfeit medicines: a real threat to the society. Int J Pharm Sci Res 2(7):1645
74. Uddin M et al (2021) Blockchain for drug traceability: architectures and open challenges. Health Informatics J 27(2):14604582211011228
75. Sahoo M, Singhar SS, Sahoo SS (2020) A blockchain based model to eliminate drug counterfeiting. Machine learning and information processing. Springer: Berlin, Germany, pp 213–222
76. Uddin M, Salah K, Jayaraman R, Pesic S, Ellahham S (2021) Blockchain for drug traceability: architectures and open challenges. Health Inform J 27(2)
77. Onderco M, Zutt M (2021) Emerging technology and nuclear security: what does the wisdom of the crowd tell us? Contemp Secur Policy, 1–26
78. Alers A et al (2019) Fundamentals of medical radiation safety: focus on reducing short-term and long-term harmful exposures. In: Vignettes in patient safety, vol 4, IntechOpen
79. Díaz M et al (2020) Integrating blockchain in safety-critical systems: an application to the nuclear industry. IEEE Access 8:190605–190619
80. Vestergaard C, Center S (2018) Blockchain and safeguards information management: the potential for distributed ledger technology. In: Symposium on international safeguards: building future safeguards capabilities
81. Yu E, Obbard E, Le L (2018) Evaluation of a blockchain based nuclear materials accounting platform in Australia. In: IAEA safeguards symposium
82. Zgierska A, Miller M, Rabago D (2012) Patient satisfaction, prescription drug abuse, and potential unintended consequences. JAMA 307(13):1377–1378
83. Raghavendra M (2019) Can Blockchain technologies help tackle the opioid epidemic: a Narrative Review. Pain Med 20(10):1884–1889
84. Om A (2018) The opioid crisis in black and white: the role of race in our nation's recent drug epidemic. J Public Health 40(4):e614–e615
85. Skolnick P (2018) On the front lines of the opioid epidemic: rescue by naloxone. Eur J Pharmacol 835:147–153
86. Reynolds W (2019) Prisoners to addiction: the forgotten victims of the 21st century opioid crisis
87. Thatcher C, Acharya S (2018) Pharmaceutical uses of blockchain technology. In: 2018 IEEE international conference on advanced networks and telecommunications systems (ANTS). IEEE
88. Adelman JS et al (2017) Evaluating serial strategies for preventing wrong-patient orders in the NICU. Pediatrics 139(5)

89. Kannampallil TG et al (2018) Effect of number of open charts on intercepted wrong-patient medication orders in an emergency department. J Am Med Inform Assoc 25(6):739–743
90. Green RA et al (2015) Intercepting wrong-patient orders in a computerized provider order entry system. Ann Emerg Med 65(6):679–686. e1
91. Tridandapani S et al (2013) Increasing rate of detection of wrong-patient radiographs: use of photographs obtained at time of radiography. Am J Roentgenol 200(4):W345–W352
92. Sandberg WS et al (2005) Automatic detection and notification of "Wrong Patient—Wrong Location" errors in the operating room. Surg Innov 12(3):253–260
93. Dunn EJ, Moga PJ (2010) Patient misidentification in laboratory medicine: a qualitative analysis of 227 root cause analysis reports in the Veterans Health Administration. Arch Pathol Lab Med 134(2):244–255
94. Esmaeilzadeh P, Mirzaei T (2019) The potential of blockchain technology for health information exchange: experimental study from patients' perspectives. J Med Int Res 21(6): N.PAG-N.PAG
95. Hylock RH, Zeng X (2019) a blockchain framework for patient-centered health records and exchange (HealthChain): evaluation and proof-of-concept study. J Med Int Res 21(8):N. PAG-N.PAG
96. Alliance SC (2003) Using smart cards for secure physical access
97. Bharatbhai-Patel S et al (2020) BioUAV: blockchain-envisioned framework for digital identification to secure access in next-generation UAVs. In: DroneCom '20: proceedings of the 2nd ACM MobiCom workshop on drone assisted wireless communications for 5G and beyond, pp 43–48
98. Rouhani S, Pourheidari V, Deters R (2018) Physical access control management system based on permissioned blockchain. In: 2018 IEEE international conference on internet of things (iThings) and IEEE green computing and communications (GreenCom) and IEEE Cyber, Physical and Social Computing (CPSCom) and IEEE Smart Data (SmartData), pp 1078–1083
99. Di Francesco Maesa D, Mori P, Ricci L (2019) A blockchain based approach for the definition of auditable access control systems. Comput Secur 84:93–119
100. Stawicki SP et al (2010) Portable ultrasonography in mass casualty incidents: The CAVEAT examination. World J Orthopedics 1(1):10
101. Wydo S et al (2016) Portable ultrasound in disaster triage: a focused review. Eur J Trauma Emerg Surg 42(2):151–159
102. Gillis J et al (2016) Panacea's cloud: Augmented reality for mass casualty disaster incident triage and co-ordination. In: 2016 13th IEEE annual consumer communications & networking conference (CCNC). IEEE
103. Ray PP, Mukherjee M, Shu L (2017) Internet of things for disaster management: state-of-the-art and prospects. IEEE Access 5:18818–18835
104. Jin H et al (2019) A review of secure and privacy-preserving medical data sharing. IEEE Access 7:61656–61669
105. Wang W et al (2021) Blockchain-assisted handover authentication for intelligent telehealth in multi-server edge computing environment. J Syst Architect 115:102024
106. Miyachi K, Mackey TK (2021) hOCBS: A privacy-preserving blockchain framework for healthcare data leveraging an on-chain and off-chain system design. Inf Process Manage 58 (3):102535
107. Alladi T et al (2019) Blockchain applications for industry 4.0 and industrial IoT: a review. IEEE Access 7:176935–176951
108. Mazumder S (2016) Big data tools and platforms. Big data concepts, theories, and applications. Springer, pp 29–128
109. Farahani B et al (2018) Towards fog-driven IoT eHealth: promises and challenges of IoT in medicine and healthcare. Futur Gener Comput Syst 78:659–676
110. Rodrigues P (2013) Large scale interoperability in the context of Future Internet. Université Sciences et Technologies-Bordeaux I

111. Salimitari M, Chatterjee M (2018) An overview of blockchain and consensus protocols for IoT networks, pp 1–12 arXiv preprint arXiv:1809.05613

112. Domnich A et al (2020) Attitudes and beliefs on influenza vaccination during the COVID-19 pandemic: results from a representative Italian survey. Vaccines 8(4):711

113. Hausman BL (2017) Immunity, modernity, and the biopolitics of vaccination resistance. Configurations 25(3):279–300

114. Penders B (2017) Vaccines, science and trust. Nat Microbiol 2(6):1–1

115. Iwasaki A, Omer SB (2020) Why and how vaccines work. Cell 183(2):290–295

116. Orenstein W (2019) Vaccines don't save lives. Vaccinations save lives. Human Vacc Immunotherapeutics 15(12):2786–2789

117. Firstenberg MS, McCallister D, Stawicki SP (2021) Insights Into a Post-COVID world. Bethlehem, Pennsylvania, USA: IllumiPress13

118. Ali MS et al (2018) Applications of blockchains in the internet of things: a comprehensive survey. IEEE Commun Surv Tutorials 21(2):1676–1717

119. Wu M et al (2019) A comprehensive survey of blockchain: From theory to IoT applications and beyond. IEEE Internet Things J 6(5):8114–8154

120. Dramé-Maigné S (2019) Blockchain and access control: towards a more secure Internet of Things. Université Paris-Saclay (ComUE)

121. Burke G, Saxena N (2021) Cyber risks prediction and analysis in medical emergency equipment for situational awareness. Sensors 21(16):5325

122. Sunhare P, Chowdhary RR, Chattopadhyay MK (2020) Internet of things and data mining: an applications oriented survey. J King Saud Univ Comput Inform Sci

123. Karimpour N et al (2019) Iot based hand hygiene compliance monitoring. In: 2019 International symposium on networks, computers and communications (ISNCC). IEEE

124. Griggs KN et al (2018) Healthcare blockchain system using smart contracts for secure automated remote patient monitoring. J Med Syst 42(7):1–7

125. Moreno HBR et al (2019) IoT in medical context: applications, diagnostics, and health care. Innovation in Medicine and Healthcare Systems, and Multimedia. Springer, pp 253–259

126. Gia TN et al (2017) IoT-based continuous glucose monitoring system: a feasibility study. Procedia Comput Sci 109:327–334

127. Rahmat MA et al (2017) GluQo: IoT-based non-invasive blood glucose monitoring. J Telecommun Electr Comput Eng (JTEC) 9(3–9):71–75

128. McBee MP, Wilcox C (2020) Blockchain technology: principles and applications in medical imaging. J Digit Imaging 33(3):726–734

129. Lucas J, Bulbul T, Thabet W (2013) An object-oriented model to support healthcare facility information management. Autom Constr 31:281–291

130. Tseng J-H et al (2018) Governance on the drug supply chain via gcoin blockchain. Int J Environ Res Public Health 15(6):1055

131. Belhi A et al (2020) Blockchains: a conceptual assessment from a product lifecycle implementation perspective. In: IFIP international conference on product lifecycle management. Springer

132. Stawicki S, Gerlach A (2009) Polypharmacy and medication errors: stop, listen, look, and analyze. Opus 12:6–10

133. Clifford GD, Clifton D (2012) Wireless technology in disease management and medicine. Annu Rev Med 63:479–492

134. Qiu Z, Zhu Y (2021) A novel structure of blockchain applied in vaccine quality control: double-chain structured blockchain system for vaccine anticounterfeiting and traceability. J Healthc Eng 2021:6660102

135. Golan MS et al (2021) The vaccine supply chain: a call for resilience analytics to support COVID-19 vaccine production and distribution. COVID-19: Systemic Risk and Resilience. Springer, pp 389–437

136. Horton E (2018) Balancing patient control and practical access policy for electronic health records via blockchain technology

137. Khezr S et al (2019) Blockchain technology in healthcare: a comprehensive review and directions for future research. Appl Sci 9(9):1736
138. Firdaus A et al (2018) Root exploit detection and features optimization: mobile device and blockchain based medical data management. J Med Syst 42(6):112
139. Kamarudin MH et al (2017) A logitboost-based algorithm for detecting known and unknown web attacks. IEEE Access 5:26190–26200
140. Lai T et al (2013) Estonia: health system review. Health Syst Transit 15(6):1–196
141. security and safety
142. Sikkut R (2019) Learning from the Estonia e-health system. Available from: https://www.healtheuropa.eu/estonian-e-health-system/89750/
143. Technology (2021). Available from: https://guardtime.com/technology
144. Healthcare (2021) [cited 2021]. Available from: https://e-estonia.com/solutions/healthcare/
145. Garrity M (2019) 4 hurdles blockchain must overcome to be mainstream

Blockchain in Medical Education

M. A. A. K. Munasinghe, M. A. S. C. Samarakoon, and M. P. P. Dilhani

Would you know the signs by which in man or an institution you may recognize old fogeyism? They are three: First a state of blissful happiness and contentment with things as they are; secondly, a supreme conviction that the condition of other people and other institutions is one of pitiable inferiority; thirdly a fear of change which not alone perplexes but appals.

—William Osler

Abstract

Medical education is a course of study directed at acquiring knowledge and skills necessary for preventing and treating disease to the aspiring students, enabling them to explore still unknown facts promoting health or causing illness. The physician thus educated has to be sensitive to needs of his setting while engaging in continuously improving knowledge and wisdom of the art and science of medicine. A blockchain is a system of digitally encrypted recording information kept in a network and a ledger of transaction that is difficult or impossible to change hack or cheat that will be invaluable as we move forward in new paradigm of medical education. Using digital encrypted network of individual student identification learner records management globally accessible medical assessment certification and validation will be made faster accurate and accessible to everyone. Funding payments educational e commerce through Blockchain makes it easier for different institutions and individuals to explore and make available services in much more streamlined and transparent manner while enhancing participation and accreditation of cpd programs. Clinical e learning will open a new vistas as securing of privacy will enable patient data

M. A. A. K. Munasinghe (✉) · M. A. S. C. Samarakoon
Ministry of Health, Sri Lanka, Colombo 10, Sri Lanka
e-mail: drakmunasinghe@gmail.com

M. P. P. Dilhani
Postgraduate Institute of Medicine, University of Colombo, Sri Lanka, Colombo 07, Sri Lanka

and and analysis to be done in multitude of centers transcending geographical boundaries. The Medical meta university conceptualized as ' entire is greater than sum of parts,'denotes significant transformation of higher education. It can explore exploit and create synergies between projects exercises and organization. Filling in as a common forum of interconnectivity. Assimilation enabling cost savings optimization of resources utility while overcoming economical and geographical constraints This will blend conventional practices with emerging breakthrough research and evidence based updates. The significant saving of time and money and improved opportunities by elimination of bogus qualifications by hitherto unavailable realtime authentication offer tremendous benefits.

Keywords

Blockchain · Digital encryption · Education · Higher education · Knowledge management · Medical education

Objectives

1. Introduction to Medical Education and Blockchain
2. Identity, learner records management and learner credential
3. Funding, payment, and educational e-commerce
4. Medical Meta University
5. Global medical assessment - Validation, Authentication and Certification
6. Clinical E-Learning
7. Medical CPD (Continued Professional Development)

Medical Education—A new paradigm

Introduction to Medical Education and Blockchain

Encyclopedia Brittanica defines Medical Education as a "course of study directed toward imparting the knowledge and skills required for the prevention and treatment of disease [to persons seeking to become physicians]. It also develops the methods and objectives appropriate to the study of the still unknown factors that produce disease or favor well-being. Among the goals of medical education is the production of physicians sensitive to the health needs of their country, capable of ministering to those needs and aware of the necessity of continuing their own education" [1] (Fig. 9.1).

The target of the clinical instruction educational plans is to offer the doctors with the ideal information and aptitudes basic to treat the patient successfully beyond expectations. Clinical Education can likewise be applied in clinical agencies preparing the executives programs [2].

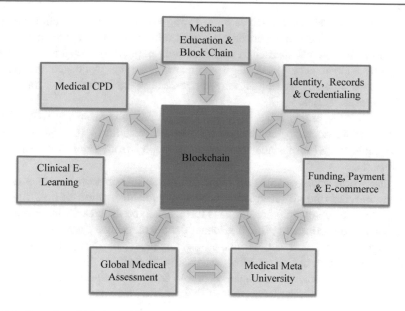

Fig. 9.1 Domains of Medical Education on the Block Chain

Until the recent past, clinical schooling comprised of homeroom addresses, notes and books with face to face instruction. The improvement in innovation and the web have supplanted the previous learning alternatives with computerized decisions, internet educating, and e-learning arrangements. The extent of clinical schooling and preparation are subject to a tremendous change with the ascent of innovation. For example, 3D Mechanism of Action, e-learning modules (Online), computer-generated experience, increased virtual reality, blended reality, email showcasing, etc. Presently these decisions incorporate as a centrepiece in many current educational plans in clinical foundations, CME programs, clinical affiliations, pharmaceuticals, healthcare organizations etc.in continued exceptional preparedness in clinics, pharmacies, labs and other clinical entities. The healthcare industry, medical education overall, are advancing rapidly with improved quality principles as an ongoing continuous process. Therefore, it is imperative that all in clinical practices needs to stay aware of the ever-changing techniques for Health Management and the related consistency guidelines.

Inability to adapt to progressing changes invariably means increased litigations, claims, and punishments. To survive, clinical practices should allocate resources to the preparation and advancement of their professionals. An advanced culture of proceeding with CME to guarantee acquiring the most recent information in their fields will empower the professionals to keep up consistency and effectiveness simultaneously enhancing the quality of care to patients.

The healthcare industry is advancing continuously in a compelling climate with feverish timetables and tremendously strict quality principles. In this manner, clinical training assumes an essential part in the turn of events and improvement of the medical services sector. E-Learning arrangements, which are effective, productive and dependable, have arisen rapidly as a favorable tool for the approval of proceeding with clinical instruction programs with improved acceptance by patients and professionals. The Medical—Healthcare Learning Management System (LMS) is one of such e-learning arrangements. These are intended for clinical and healthcare associations.

By picking the proper LMS for preparing in clinical consistency will enhance harmony among doctors, patients and the healthcare industry in a more comprehensive manner and also shield medical care faculty from expensive claims and punishments.

As the world changes to being more informed, information becomes another currency moving into an information economy and information life. At the same time, protection of key common liberties turns out to be progressively hard to keep up in its present context. With the idea of web of things characterized as "an organization of physical and virtual articles, gadgets, or things that are fit for gathering encompassing information and trading it starting them or through the web" and applications, for example, wearable individual wellbeing trackers, purchasers are turning into the focal point of their very own consideration management [3].

With the above idea, a significant issue emerges that is information protection and security. The answer lies in comprehending the idea of square chain, which can be characterized as "A route for individuals to take care of issues by sharing things" [4].

The idea of blockchain will have an incredible effect and will be a game-changer in future comparable to the internet of things including artificial intelligence. "Blockchain has been alluded to as the biggest mechanical and business upheaval as the approach of the Internet." Blockchain's development has emerged due to the uplifted security, tampering proof transactions, better control and accessability to information. Blockchain is an innovation that considers secure storage, correspondence, and trade of information [5].

Blockchain is made out of individual blocks. Each block contains data to be put away; a hash, which is a security key that particularly distinguishes the data in that block, and a record of the hash on the past block in the chain. In the event that any one block is altered, the hash or unique mark of that block changes. When this happens, all resulting blocks in the chain become mindful of the altering as the hash of the altered block no longer matches past records. By connecting the blocks in this style into a chain, altering gets almost impossible (Fig. 9.2).

Blockchain permits its approved members to see and confirm all the information and exchanges contained in any one block of the chain, where those are checked and scrambled prior to being added to the block diminishing odds of misrepresentation. This can be recognized as a critical element of blockchain idea where so that a programmer would have to have dramatically more processing ability to break in than is needed in the present different frameworks. Additionally, once information exchanges are on a block, they can't be overwritten, and no focal organization holds control, as these records are obvious to all the clients associated

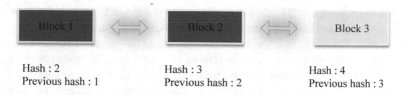

Hash : 2   Hash : 3   Hash : 4
Previous hash : 1   Previous hash : 2   Previous hash : 3

Fig. 9.2 Blocks in Blockchain

with them. Clients' characters inside a record are known uniquely to the clients themselves.

Blockchain is most popular as the innovation supporting Bitcoin and other cryptographic forms of money. The basic innovation, notwithstanding, which uses progressed software engineering to keep up secure, conveyed information records, has far more extensive expected uses and is now being embraced across a few businesses, including mining and common assets, food industry etc. Medical care also will profit by propels in blockchain innovation, with the potential for it to affect the consideration of patients, just as the credentialing of clinical experts [6].

Deliberately, blockchain offers ways for "individuals who don't know or trust each other to make a record of who owns what." As a method of making and ensuring trust, it has expansive ramifications past monetary [7]. Blockchain saddles the force of encryption to attest its own permanence and become a more secure choice than any actual information base. Blockchain places the patient at the focal point of the medicalcare environment more than some other frameworks [8].

Zhang, Douglas, Schmidt, and White [9] identified the following seven uses for blockchain in healthcare:

(a) Prescription tracking to detect opioid overdose and over-prescription
(b) Data sharing to incorporate telemedicine with traditional care
(c) Sharing cancer data with providers using patient authorized access
(d) Cancer registry sharing to aggregate observations in cancer cases
(e) Management of patient digital identity for better patient record matching
(f) Personal health records for accessing and controlling complete health history
(g) Adjudication automation of health insurance claims to surface error and fraud.

Blockchain's incentive in medical services stretches beyond security and protection allowing common access to health-related data for clinicians, healthcare facilities, and patients [10]. Its utilization can bring about expanded clinician time for persistent consideration, sharing of research and developments in new medicines, and upgraded best practices. Minimization of guarantee and charging misrepresentation is another benefit with simplified admittance to their medicalcare records empowering patients to share their records with other medicalcare experts in a consistent, time-compelling way.

Most drastically, blockchain can change clinical development—and maybe even forecast and anticipation of malignancy. An individual's genomic information holds high prognostication value, especially corresponding to endeavors to improve outcome in malignancy [11]. In 2018, one start-up that used blockchain innovation declared an association with a main atomic diagnostics organization to quicken the forecast of malignant growth for many people around the world [12]. Subsequently, most current information from everywhere in the world in medication can be shared in a split second in a reliable way by utilizing this blockchain framework.

Blockchain stands to alter how we track clinical schooling, confirm competence, and authentication of clinical experts, a cycle that has become extremely taxing and unwieldy for clinicians and establishments as well. As a worldwide application the potential of this is gigantic. Blockchains could improve clinical instruction and credentialing universally, and empower another epoc of streamlining regulation of professionalism.

Medical education transcends geographical boundaries with an added advantage to dependably track, vet and check learning and teaching modules and institutional objectives through blockchain. The students will be uniquely identified and their progress will be recorded through a secure and time logged system with all their clinical experiences, learning modules, practical involvements catalogued. Even the depth of each scenario, intended learning outcomes, degree of compliance could be tracked from anywhere. This forms a complete ecosystem where clinicians, patients, other stakeholders and different institutions independently verify and evaluate a student's performance. For those specialities that rely on hands-on training and skills, it will be an added bonus with an assessment of technical strengths and weaknesses can convert to tailor-made training schedule for an individual recruited. In research, it would result in better collaborations, originalities rather than duplicates.

CME will possess an added meaning as the career pathway redefines with time-stamped certifications of college memberships and affiliations with activities logged. Involvements in publications, research, teaching, training and conference attendance will be updated and validated real-time. However, the flipside is litigations, lawsuits, diciplinary breaches too will be visible on the same resume (Fig. 9.3).

Identity, Learner Records Management and Learner Credentialing

Globally there is no regular framework to confirm clinical certifications or licenses. International credentialing measures are generally tedious and costly as providers require record keeping and clerical work in different methodologies and varied languages. The issuing authorities everywhere in the world need interoperability as its essential yield is a comprehensive authorized transcript [6].

Associations invest significant amount of resources on validation of scholastic certifications [13–16]. By granting academic certifications on a blockchain, a definite, clear and time stamped record can be issued [17]. In the event of lost records (migrants/asylum clinical students/specialists with no permitance to their respective

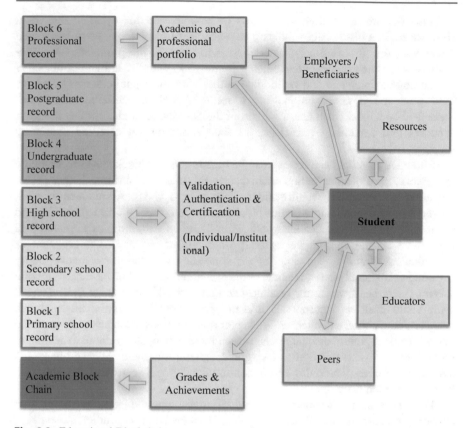

Fig. 9.3 Educational Blockchain

organization) or a specialist/clinical student moving to different licensing authorities, a record on the blockchain is readily accessible around the world without the need for a separate transcript from the issuing authority [18]. The information is cryptographically encoded, and only the individuals who have the computerized keys can access the accreditations.

Illustration

A specialist from nation 'X' gets his clinical recognition on a blockchain. He claims and controls the "private keys" to his blockchain account. He moves to the nation 'Y' subsequent to turning into a displaced person. The Medical Council in the nation 'Y' can't contact his parent foundation. Since the 'hash'—the novel computerized stamp of his degree is given on a blockchain, the record is autonomously undeniable. He later applies for enrollment with the Medical Council in nation 'Y' which had the option to freely confirm his qualifications without wanting to counsel the first foundation in nation 'X'.

Initiatives are as of now in progress to smooth out this cycle in the USA. HashedHealth, a blockchain wellbeing advancement organization, as of late joined forces with the Illinois Blockchain Initiative to improve the proficiency and precision of the state's clinical credentialing framework, with the drawn out objective of rearranging interstate and multi state authorizing on a public scale. Likewise, Intel proposed a novel outline for a multi-layered credentialing framework dependent on a blockchain that would profit the two doctors and clinics by reducing expenses and expanding proficiency of this 'upsetting yet essential regulatory capacity' [6].

Instructive materials and records can be transferred to a blockchain credentialing framework, a protected online archive, would make a uniform language for preparing accreditations, confirmations, degrees and CME. Admittance to one's instructive and expert history on this blockchain would then be able to be safely and promptly imparted to credentialing offices utilizing an extraordinary computerized key where all the appropriate material are recorded in detail. Confirmation of accreditations could happen either by the conceding foundation (ie, a college), by checking establishments (ie, medical clinic credentialing workplaces or authorizing sheets), a service of wellbeing, or almost certain a mix of these. Each fruitful check cycle could itself be incorporated into the permanent blockchain, lessening the danger of fake action and altering. Whenever qualifications are checked by confided in organizations, future credentiarlers can see those safe cycles without expecting to re-confirm each accreditation at its source, saving suppliers the exorbitant and tedious cycle of re-mentioning and re-communicating their certifications with each new expert open door.

Blockchain stands to make a record of one's schooling and preparing that encourages credentialing. When a supplier is credentialed or authorized training blockchain can additionally smooth out upkeep of confirmation through concentrated CME following. Courses taken, gatherings joined in, papers and books read, proficient system logs, or some other scholastic exercises could be naturally fused into a supplier's credentialing blockchain—permitting a quick, obvious, and permanent instruction record for looking after affirmation, authorizing, and proficient progression. Blockchain could bind together the whole 'instructive life expectancy' of clinicians into one changeless, straightforward, worldwide, and evident record (Fig. 9.4).

Funding, Payment, and Educational E-commerce

Clinical training "tokens" can be made on a decentralized Blockchain which can be utilized to pay for instructive administrations straightforwardly from a portable wallet. This will empower end clients to associate straightforwardly with the schooling specialist organizations and permit them to pay for instructive administrations in computerized money [19].

Fig. 9.4 Blockchain in
Identity, learner records
management and
credentialing

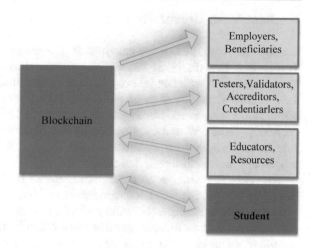

The computerized tokens could likewise be granted for scholastic accomplishments which can be acknowledged as an acknowledgment of grant by various foundations based on a pre-concurred models. A blockchain based stage will permit clients to look, associate, and pay for instructive administrations in a self-supporting online business eco-framework that will be around the world available in all nations that allows its tasks inside their administrative structure [20]. An advanced passage will permit instructive offices to deal with understudy's data, prizes, and support in instructive exercises in a more smoothed out way.

Illustration

- Empower foundations to enlist as Education Service Providers and auto-execute shrewd agreements dependent on pre-concurred sets of standards [21]
- Publicize scholarly courses, gatherings, distributions, projects, books, magazine, diary, research article, classes, instructional exercises, addresses, workshops to a worldwide blockchain local area
- Quest for administrations by classification, control or guide and book straightforwardly by means of blockchain installment entryway without the need of a delegate
- Boost the makers of instructive substance as computerized tokens or declarations conveyed shared, without the need of a confided in outsider
- Alternative to share instructive substance via online media straightforwardly from a blockchain entryway
- Alternatives to rate coaches, courses and foundations progressively and share the input with numerous partners
- Associate and offer information with everybody associated with the blockchain eco-framework, profiting by an affectionate, worldwide clinical organization.

Medical Meta University

Charles M. Vest, president—emeritus at America's Massachusetts Institute of Technology, first discussed the rise of the meta-college in a discourse in 2006. Nonetheless, if completely realized India could be host to the world's first public meta-college [22]. The idea of Meta University permits a student to profit by admittance to academics, library and research centers of different institutions while pursuing a degree. With the appearance of this framework, students would now be able to be registered for a credit transfer framework between colleges offering adaptability and multi-faculty training.

The Meta University conceptualized as 'Entire is Greater than the Sum of the Parts', denotes a significant transformation in Higher Education. It can explore, exploit and create synergies between projects, exercises and organizations filling in as a common forum of interconnectivity and assimiliation enabling the best use of resources minimizing the costs and economical and geographical constraints. Additionally, this initiative synchronises the best in conventional practices with novel vistas offering greater possibilities to all associates with added advantages:

- New program
- Flexible platforms
- Greater access
- Wider assimilation
- Enhanced synchronization
- Promote creativity
- Innovations for critical thinking

Key components

- Makes another worldview in information frameworks
- Dependence on National Knowledge Network
- Pooling of assets by various organizations
- Formation of collaborations in creative projects
- Utilization of data innovation for virtual learning
- Development in information procurement
- Consolidating "Synergistic learning" and "Trans-disciplinary learning"
- Guide to fill in as the Catalyst

Topographically separated a few foundations can consolidate so as to give the understudies some hypothetical sources of info and significant active involvement with information making in the field of medication. The Degree course will mirror a trans-disciplinary methodology and will advance new perspectives, making the learning and showing measure happy and beneficial. Out of a few encouraging stages including study hall, virtual and project based learning, blockchain framework would be the best method to make the meta college idea a triumph. Intuitive strategies for guidance will be empowered. Understudies will take mixes of courses from the accomplice foundations where they are accessible on-line on squares.

Undertakings will be given fundamental significance and coaches will assume key part in gathering project work. Guides will be painstakingly chosen for their aptitude in the significant regions. They might be from both inside the accomplice organizations and outside where all are associated by the blockchain framework.

Learning in a clinical climate is progressively perplexing and can be hard to record [23]. It is regularly a genuine test to diagram of program and self-coordinated learning [24]. Clinical understudies and specialists learn tremendous measures of information and abilities that are hard to reflect, confirm, recognize and approve [25]. Regularly, it is practically difficult to follow the learning back to each and every source. Since the approval on blockchain happens at the hour of production of a record and not a while later, a blockchain based program could offer an answer for this difficult difficulty. It is presently for all intents and purposes workable for instructive substance to be scrambled, approved, time stepped and made accessible on a blockchain. Instructive substance is changelessly put away on a decentralized record [26]. The student can get to the information from anyplace on the planet and give moment criticism to the maker by "hash labeling" the applicable pieces of data. This will at that point be credited to the maker's portfolio in a totally decentralized, lasting, sealed type of proof. A framework dependent on blockchain will likewise recognize commitment to the general public when all is said in done which would somehow have not been conceivable—an arrangement of instruction that removes the action from the customary domains of organizations to a totally worldwide, all around available environment. Cryptography would guarantee straightforwardness, perceivability and complete client control in a shared manner without the need of a confided in mediator.

Illustration

A clinical understudy goes to nation 'Z' on a position where he invests energy locally accomplishing charitable effort. He additionally goes through about fourteen days all in all training and seven days in the lab. Since the learning log is available on a blockchain based PDA, appraisals and reflections can be put away progressively on a lasting record. Assessors can give contemporaneous input which can be carefully put away on the blockchain. The log book of arrangement would then be able to be partaken in a private way with the assessors and college staff. Every section is time stepped, autonomously evident and forever recorded on the understudy's college document [27] (Fig. 9.5).

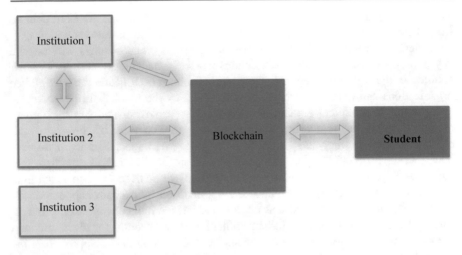

Fig. 9.5 Blockchain and Meta University

Global Medical Assessment—Validation, Authentication, and Certification

The blast of phony degrees and associations that produce them (named by numerous individuals as "certificate factories") has made a ton of vulnerability in the scholastic space as well as the public's trust of experts. This developing issue with counterfeit accreditations sabotages the very texture of higher learning as it deteriorates the time, difficult work and basic incentive chasing advanced education. Shockingly, there are grave contrasts when we are talking about how individuals see the authenticity between the business and clinical fields. It is one thing for there to be doubt of the President of Microsoft China [28], yet it is a lot of more regrettable if individuals begin to question the capacities of their clinical experts. This can prompt an entire host of concerns, for example, patients not adhering to guidelines with respect to sedate admission, restoration or numerous others and afterward turning to accuse the absence of trust in the guardian as the purpose behind their proceeding with issues or sicknesses. People with counterfeit degrees put general society in danger as their expressed range of abilities is missing because of negligible information or a total nonattendance of preparing. Some venture to such an extreme as to utilize their fake certifications to acquire individuals' trust and afterward misuse it to sell self-composed scam on the web and bait patients from genuine drug. This is actually what happened when two men who bought their PCPs' ID's for $100 took a little youngster off insulin who kicked the bucket subsequent to taking their mixture [29]. They were therefore accused of homicide in North Carolina.

This issue has existed for quite a long time yet as of late detonated in the previous few decades to a great extent because of advances in innovation. Maybe the most well known late illustration of far and wide maltreatment includes the Axact organization in Pakistan concocting more than 300 phony colleges and utilizing created reports to trick businesses who may check references. Axact's CEO and 22 representatives got 20-year sentences each for their phony degree plant [30]. That may appear to be enormous, however it could not hope to compare with regards to the new blast of this in China over the most recent ten years. The issue has become so broad that there are sites being made trip these cheats alongside "valid or bogus" gateways where clients can check schools not recorded. China's service of schooling has been effectively focusing on crackdowns too.

It has additionally been seen where people acting like clinical experts are instructing with their "doctored" doctorates [31]. At University of Victoria, Mr. Jason Matthew Walker trained courses in kid and youth care in 2006. This subverts the school required as well as imperils the authenticity of the levels of the under-studies being instructed. He later turned into a chief of private administrations at Glengarry Hospital. The representative for the Vancouver Island Health Authority Shannon Marshall expressed "We wouldn't regularly check the certifications of any lesser of center chief except if there was some sign they should have been con-firmed". When an individual is gotten with ill-conceived degrees it isn't generally a simple cycle to attempt to translate the number of the degrees this individual professes to hold are genuine and the number of are just purchased on the web.

Previous FBI specialist Allen Ezell claims over portion of the PhDs gave in the United States each year are phony [31] and subtleties this marvel broadly in the book he co-composed Degree Mills: The Billion Dollar Industry that has sold over 1,000,000 phony certificates. The phony recognition market goes back similarly as the fourteenth century in Europe [32] and of the assessed 200,000 phony certificates for each year gave by factories situated in the United States alone, a sizable segment is assessed to be "granted" to those in the clinical field.

Utilizing the different blockchain techniques point by point above, we accept this could be the response to a centuries old issue that is getting considerably more inescapable with time. The measure of work, energy and cash exhausted by people attempting to battle this developing issue could be saved by making open and straightforward blockchain scholarly declarations that truly mirror the genuine work used by the understudy.

Clinical E-Learning

One can start to see a future for training that offers understudies a great help inside which they create applicable information, comprehension, and abilities at a serious cost and with successful and effective instructive techniques. The instructive vehicle should be helpful for understudies, advancing adaptability and empowering the understudies to concentrate anyplace advantageous, time permitting, with non-compromising self evaluation.

The instructive system will challenge understudies with issues that are proto-typical instances of the scope of pathophysiological measures while simultaneously underscoring those conditions that are regular in the local area. Issues will reference a wide scope of literary and varying media materials, all completely listed for multi-hub looking and available on the web. Understudies will peruse and look through these assets to find intriguing data, investigating virtual anatomical, histological, clinical, careful, and neurotic examples, pictures, and techniques on their PC in shading and with three dimensional appearance.

Interest in structures and study halls for study will be diminished, as will the need to eliminate understudies for extensive stretches from their local area to focuses of the scholarly community. The requirement for actual admittance to materials, for example, dead bodies, examples, and diary articles will be to a great extent disposed of. Intuitive, ease web meetings will connect specialists with understudies in various areas. Programming will "serve" the progressive segments of a course straightforwardly to the understudies when and where they may require it.

By and large, the likely exists to incredibly decrease costs while offering understudies a "administration" that is adaptable, advantageous, and productive and can be custom fitted to meet precisely their own necessities and conditions. In wide terms similar standards ought to apply to concentrate after graduation.

Arrangement of understudies to experience with patients may include intelligent reproductions, models, and PC based test systems. The procurement of certain abilities will at present require apprenticeship, for example, figuring out how to cooperate with and inspect patients and to perform actual methodology and creating humanistic and caring perspectives. These abilities can be gained any place there are skilled consideration suppliers capable and ready to bestow them. Surely, at present understudies are dispatched to different areas of essential and optional consideration on connections, revolutions, and electives to build up these aptitudes similarly. As far as we can tell a portion of these abilities, and especially the mentalities, might be better moved by good examples from the focuses of academe.

The significant issue is to guarantee that understudies have grown fittingly, which should be done through appraisals of wellness to rehearse in moderately customary manners and under controlled and managed conditions.

- 3D imaging of the inside organs

The ascent in innovation and improvement in 3D picture advancement programming have empowered the clinical specialists to imagine your interior organs through the computerized framework. This is of colossal significance as before it was impractical to know the specific situation of the interior organs and how they are working or adjusted without getting along any pragmatic on gave dead bodies. You can likewise imagine inconsistencies in patient bodies through 3D pictures.

- Utilization of computer generated reality in clinical industry

The clinical business is perhaps the biggest connector of the recently evolved vivid innovation, augmented reality. This incorporates reproduction of medical procedure, automated tasks, therapy of fear, system of activity, therapy modalities, understanding case and clinical preparing. This innovation has a great favorable position that it empowers the experts to revive their aptitudes while learning the new ones and the progression in clinical treatment. Augmented reality has numerous applications in the clinical business, from the advancement of new life-saving strategies to preparing future doctors.

- Communicating through the web with the subject matter experts and writing for a blog

The clinical online club has grown colossally with the coming of web-based media. Content improvement for courses is encouraged by the accessibility of e-learning assets making things a lot simpler. Experts in Healthcare need to stay aware of the most recent endorsements in expert turn of events and related permitting. Diverse Exam Master offers a wide scope of assessment addresses which at last produce better analysts. A positive presentation and inspiration reaction to e-learning has been shown by a few specialists.

- SkillPort: Another cloud-based arrangement

This cloud-based learning the executives framework empowers the clients of the e-learning courses and projects to follow, oversee, and report their advancement. The arrangement offers commonly planned courses through instructional booklets, digital books, and recordings and furthermore offers affirmation preparing.

- Preventive consideration courses

In practically every emergency clinic and center, e-learning arrangements are advancing with progressing credit-based courses accessible for all the doctor and paramedics. For example, a moderately new control known as palliative consideration program has begun in wellbeing communities through e-Learning offices. The course gives tips to care for fundamentally sick or biting the dust family members and how to deal with the stun and life after their demise. Likewise, the learning the board framework can assist with sharing encounters for diabetes patients, drunkards, and smokers.

- Enlarged Reality Medical Education

Among the main patterns in Medical Education and Medical Technology, medical care enlarged reality legitimately takes a main position. With more than 1 billion clients it opens a pool of chances for medical care and drug ventures. Enlarged reality in clinical schooling can fill various needs. It assists the students with obtaining, measure, and recall the clinical data. Moreover, Healthcare Augmented Reality makes learning itself additionally captivating and fun.

Medical CPD (Continued Professional Development)

Proceeding with Medical Education (CME) alludes to a particular type of training framework for doctors that comprises of various instructive and expert exercises. These exercises serve to create, keep up, and increment the information, aptitudes, proficient execution and connections that a doctor or a specialist uses to offer types of assistance for their patients, general society, or the calling. Each CME movement has a specific number of credits related with it called CME credits. Each specialist needs to acquire a base number of CME credits to restore their clinical permit [33].

Specialists are deep rooted students. CME programs have encouraged a culture among specialists to get refreshed with the most recent advancements in their claim to fame and in a roundabout way improve medical care on the planet. Likewise, a doctor's Medical License should be restored after finish of a given residency.

Clinical instruction is quickly advancing and is turning out to be progressively multidisciplinary. Clinical understudies and specialists are progressively needed to gather a wide scope of CPD joining both clinical and non-clinical exercises [34]. The blockchain can gather constant proof of realizing, which can be put away and shared immediately with the significant bodies [35]. It will likewise make it time and asset successful to screen participation records, delivering CPD endorsements on the blockchain and catching simultaneous student input. Moreover, this is of fantastic incentive in reaffirmation of student's responsibility for records and the CPD [36].

Illustration

A CPD occasion coordinator enlists all members on the blockchain. The admittance to the whole program of exercises is accessible on the blockchain. Members check the "QR code" of every introduction at the hour of enlisting their participation. Through a decentralized portable application (DApps), constant input is submitted both to the moderator and coordinator's records.

Since the endorsement of support is additionally given to the participants on a blockchain, there are critical expense and time investment funds both to the members and the coordinators. The CPD "reflection" is recorded on the blockchain which can be associated with the student's portfolio continuously (Fig. 9.6).

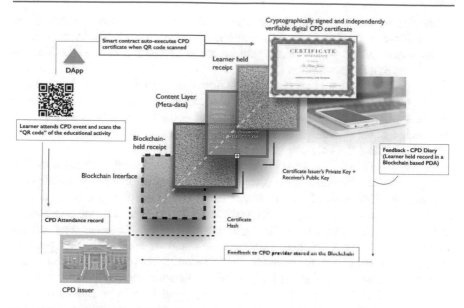

Fig. 9.6 (*Source* Copyrights Naqvi, N 2018, The British Blockchain Association) IDEALISTIC SOLUTION DESIGN—A 360 degree complete CPD Loop. Technology stack: Blockchain based CPD, Certification and Feedback

To enlist, all the current specialists will present their subtleties to the Concerning administering body. The body would check the subtleties from its current information base. On the off chance that the subtleties put together by the specialist are discovered to be right, the body would store all the subtleties related with the specialist on Inter Planetary Files System (IPFS), a convention that utilizes a novel distributed organization document sharing framework. It endeavors to address the inadequacies of Client-Server model just as that of HTTP web. Information stockpiling on IPFS if profoundly secure as it denies any alterations. It utilizes a successful method where a remarkable identifier is produced cryptographically [37], and changing the substance of information changes the identifier itself. It utilizes Distributed Hash Tables where the identifier is the key and information put away is the worth. The primary bit of leeway of utilizing IPFS for the current application is that this identifier could be put away on the decentralized application to diminish both the comprehensive computational tasks and the measure of information move over the blockchain. At that point another wallet for the specialist would be made creating a remarkable location along these lines enlisting the specialist. The utilization of IPFS for this work will help guarantee security of client information and makes the framework more productive.

Like the enrollment of Doctors, the coordinator of the occasion should present all the necessary subtleties of the Organizer to the Concerning overseeing body. When the body has gotten the subtleties, it would take the necessary choices on if to endorse the association dependent on if the association fulfills all the standards referenced by the body. On the off chance that the association is affirmed, its subtleties would be put away on the IPFS. Like the enlistment of specialists, a wallet record of the association would be made creating a remarkable location hence enrolling the association [38].

Before the occasion starts, the coordinator would need to enlist the occasion which it means to have by presenting the occasion's subtleties to the concerned overseeing body. The subtleties of the occasion would be put away in the IPFS producing a novel hash and in this way enlisting the occasion. The body would give this IPFS hash of the occasion to the coordinator (Fig. 9.7).

When the specialist has gone to the occasion, he would need to examine the QR code gave toward the finish of the occasion by the coordinator. The QR code would contain the IPFS hash of the occasion. After examining the QR code, a keen agreement would be summoned which would verify the specialist, the coordinator, and whether the association is the legitimate host of the occasion. After all the subtleties have been confirmed, a declaration would be created for the specialist indicating the subtleties, for example, the location of coordinator, address of the specialist, season of issue, the IPFS hash of the occasion and the quantity of CME credits related with the occasion. Another exceptional ID will be created for each testament gave. The subtleties of the authentication can be followed utilizing the one of a kind ID. After checking the QR code the exchange would continue on the organization just if the area of the examining gadget of the specialist is equivalent to

Fig. 9.7 Entity Registration Diagram of Proposed CME Credits system

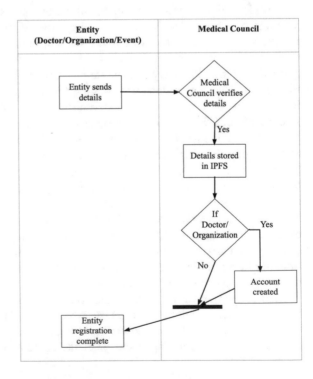

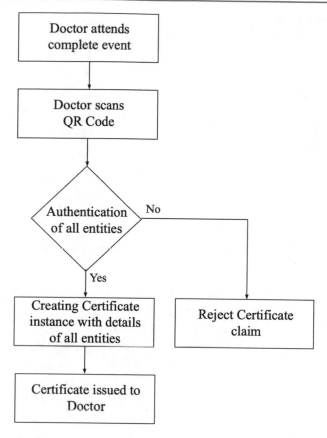

Fig. 9.8 Accreditation of CME Credits to Doctor

the area of the occasion. This will help stop the illegal utilization of the QR code to procure CME credits.(Fig. 9.8).

After every reestablishment period set by the clinical board, a savvy agreement would be consequently summoned which would check the quantity of credits gathered by the specialist utilizing the record addresses. In the event that the specialist fulfills the base CME credits prerequisite, at that point the credits related with his gathered testaments would be invalidated and their permit would be recharged. On the off chance that a specialist neglects to gather the necessary number of credits, at that point appropriate move would be made relying upon the laws of the Medical Council as talked about previously (Fig. 9.9).

At the point when a substance (Doctor, Organizer or Event) applies for enrollment, it ought to send the accompanying information to the concerned clinical committee [39]. The information referenced in the underneath table which is presented by the substance may shift contingent upon the necessities of the concerned clinical board. The clinical chamber would store all the information of the

Fig. 9.9 License Renewal
Activity

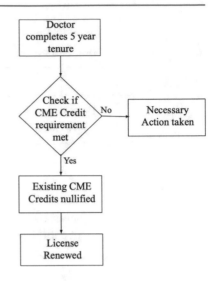

Table 9.1 Required details of entities for CME credits accreditation and license renewal

Doctor	Organization	Event
Name	Name	Organizer
Registration Number	Registration Number	Number of Speakers
Medical Council	Contact Information	Level of Event
Father's Name		Duration (in hours)
		List of delegates

substances in the IPFS and get an interesting hash that can be utilized to get to the information put away in the IPFS. On the off chance that the element to be enrolled is a Doctor or an occasion, The Concerned Medical Council would first summoned which would plan the location of the record with the comparing IPFS hash. This would communicate an exchange to the blockchain expressing that the substance has been enlisted with the given record address and IPFS hash. The Table 9.1 shows the necessary subtleties of elements.

On the off chance that the element to be enlisted is an occasion, the clinical board would initially survey all the given information of the occasion and in the event that it coordinates its necessities, at that point it would relegate a specific number of CME credits to it dependent on the rules of the separate clinical committee. At that point a savvy agreement would be conjured which would initially confirm that the coordinator of the occasion is substantial and afterward map the IPFS hash of the occasion with the location of the coordinator and the CME credits relegated to it. This will communicate an exchange to the blockchain that a given occasion with a specific association and with a particular number of CME credits is enrolled. The IPFS hash of the occasion will be given to the coordinator by the Council as QR code.

At the point when a specialist has now finished going to the occasion, They should filter a QR code which would be given toward the finish of the occasion. Checking the QR code would consequently summon a keen agreement which would initially confirm all the subtleties of the specialist, coordinator and the occasion. At that point it would produce a declaration with an interesting ID and allot it to the specialist by filling the subtleties appeared in the figure. The agreement would likewise monitor the ID's of declaration appointed to each specialist, the ID's of testament given by the coordinator and the addresses of specialist going to a specific occasion. This would communicate an exchange to the blockchain that the endorsement with a given ID has been given to the specialist by a specific association.

When the recharging time frame referenced by the separate clinical gathering gets more than, a shrewd agreement is consequently summoned which first checks whether the given specialist is substantial. In the event that the specialist is substantial it figures the quantity of CME credits gathered by them by emphasizing through the rundown of the multitude of testaments gathered by the specialist. In the event that the specialist isn't suspended and the quantity of credits gathered by them meets the necessities of the chamber then the credits related with their endorsements is invalidated and the permit of the specialist is recharged. Else on the off chance that the specialist neglects to meet the prerequisites of the gathering, at that point they are forced a fine or are suspended or some other reasonable move is made against them dependent on the guidelines determined by the concerning clinical chamber to which the specialist is related with. Regardless the exchange is communicated to the organization that the specialist with a particular IPFS hash and record address has restored their permit or a specific move has been made against them.

"Ever since Homo sapiens was evolved into his current status, medical education would have been in practice albeit in a subtle manner. In short blockchain based medical education is an Art and a science which was tempered in flames but finally sealed with kiss...."

By AM.

References

1. Gregg A (2020) Scarborough, harold and turner. Edward Lewis. Medical education. Encyclopedia Britannica [Internet]. https://www.britannica.com/science/medical-education. Available from: https://www.britannica.com/science/medical-education
2. Moisaka Solutions 3 Comments. Top 10 medical education & healthcare learning management system (2019). http://moisaka.com/top-10-medical-education-healthcare-learning-management-system/
3. Sembroiz D, Ricciardi S, Careglio D (2017) a novel cloud-based iot architecture for smart building automation. Secur resil intell data-centric syst commun networks, 215–33
4. Engelhardt MA (2017) Hitching healthcare to the chain: an introduction to blockchain technology in the healthcare sector. Technol Innov Manag Rev [Internet] 7(10). Available from: http://timreview.ca/article/1111

5. Hughes F, Morrow MJ (2019) Blockchain and health care. Policy Polit Nurs Pract 20(1):4–7
6. Can blockchain disrupt health education, licensing, and credentialling. Lancet Glob Heal Blog [Internet] (2018). Available from: https://els-jbs-prod-cdn.jbs.elsevierhealth.com/pb-assets/ Lancet/langlo/TLGH_Blogs_2013-2018-1552323974250.pdf
7. The Economist (2015) The great chain of being sure about things. Econ, 21–4
8. Koo Lalmb (2014) A blockchain for health care, 1–10
9. Zhang P, Schmidt D, White J, Lenz G, Chapter one-blockchain technology use, cases in healthcare. Adv Comput 111:1–41. https://doi.org/10.1016/bs.adcom.2018.03.006
10. Marr B (2017) This is why blockchains will transform healthcare. Forbes. https://www.forbes. com/sites/bernardmarr/2017/11/29/this-is-why-blockchains-will-transform-healthcare/#5e91c 8e11ebe
11. Scott M (2018) What can blockchain technology mean for cancer prediction and prevention. https://www.nasdaq.com/article/what-can-blockchain-technology-mean-for-cancer-prediction- and-prevention-cm933364
12. PRNewswire. Shivom partnership with genetic technologies will enable better cancer prediction and prevention through mass genomic data analysis. Retrieved from https://www. prnewswire.com/news-releases/shivom-partnership-with-genetic-technologies-will-enable- better-cancerprediction-and-prevention-through-mass-genomic-dataanalysis-675989513.html
13. Yusuf SJ (2017) Blockchain technology & healthcare credentialing: an introduction. Natl Assoc Med Staff Serv 4(April):9–15
14. Sotos J, Houlding D (2017) Blockchains for physician credentialing. Intel Corp [Internet]. Available from: https://simplecore.intel.com/itpeernetwork/wp-content/uploads/sites/38/2017/ 05/Intel_Blockchain_Application_Note2.pdf
15. Holmes L (2017) Distributed ledger technologies for public good : leadership , collaboration and innovation. House of Lords [Internet], 33. Available from: http://chrisholmes.co.uk/wp- content/uploads/2017/11/Distributed-Ledger-Technologies-for-Public-Good_leadership- collaboration-and-innovation.pdf
16. How much money do businesses spend annually on background checks? (2017) https://www. quora.com/How-much-money-do-businesses-spend-annually-on-background-checks
17. True T (2018) How will blockchain technology affect higher education in the future ? [Internet]. Openaccessgovernment.org/how-blockchain-technology-affects-higher-education/ 54512/. 2018. pp 1–5. Available from: openaccessgovernment.org/how-blockchain- technology-affects-higher-education/54512/
18. Loo B (2016) Recognizing refugee qualifications: practical tips for credential assessment
19. Naqvi N, Hussain M (2018) Medical education on the blockchain. J Br Blockchain Assoc. 1:1
20. James FJ (2018) What happens when you combine blockchain and education? https:// hackernoon.com/what-happens-when-you-combine-blockchain-and-education-d533ef6d4862
21. Watters A (2016) The blockchain for education: an introduction [Internet]. http:// hackeducation.com/2016/04/07/blockchain-education-guide. Available from: http:// hackeducation.com/2016/04/07/blockchain-education-guide
22. Mishra A (2011) INDIA: "Meta-university" plan to boost innovation. https://www. universityworldnews.com/post.php?story=20111125212118764
23. Hays R (2006) Teaching and learning in clinical settings. Radcliffe Publishing
24. Jossberger H, Brand-Gruwel S, Boshuizen H, van de Wiel M (2010) The challenge of self- directed and self-regulated learning in vocational education: a theoretical analysis and synthesis of requirements. J Vocat Educ Train [Internet] 62(4):415–40. Available from: https://doi.org/10.1080/13636820.2010.523479
25. Kristiansson MH, Troein M, Brorsson A (2014) We lived and breathed medicine—then life catches up: medical students' reflections. BMC Med Educ [Internet] 14:66. Available from: https://pubmed.ncbi.nlm.nih.gov/24690405
26. Morshed J (2017) What blockchain could mean for higher education. https://edtechnology.co. uk/Article/what-blockchain-could-mean-for-higher-ed

27. Hamilton M (2017) Blockchain in research and education. https://www.jisc.ac.uk/reports/blockchain-in-research-and-education
28. How blockchain can stamp out fake diplomas (2017). https://www.forbes.com/sites/lamsharon/2017/10/08/how-blockchain-can-stamp-out-chinas-fake-diplomas/#6cc5a6636854
29. Gibson K (2017) Your MD may have a phony degree. https://www.cbsnews.com/news/your-md-may-have-a-phony-degree/
30. Asad M (2018) Axact CEO, 22 others sentenced to 20 years in jail in fake degrees case. https://www.dawn.com/news/1418156
31. Jackson M (2017) How easy is it to fake it as a doctor? https://www.bbc.com/news/uk-40861475
32. Clarke B.B.C. doctor accused of fake credentials (2010). https://www.theglobeandmail.com/news/british-columbia/bc-doctor-accused-of-fake-credentials/article4301066/
33. Miller LA, Chen X, Srivastava V, Sullivan L, Yang W, Yii C (2015) CME credit systems in three developing countries: China, India and Indonesia. J Eur C [Internet] 4(1):27411. Available fromhttps://doi.org/10.3402/jecme.v4.27411
34. Continuing Professional Development (2017) Clin experiment ophthalmol 45(6):658–9
35. Korzhova IV (2019) Blockchain in education. Qual Innov Educ, 32–35
36. Acheson N (2017) Blockchain and education: a big idea in need of bigger thinking. https://www.coindesk.com/blockchain-education-big-idea-need-bigger-thinking
37. Vuji\vcić D, Jagodić D, Rao_ić S (2018) Blockchain technology, bitcoin, and Ethereum: a brief overview. 2018 17th international symposium INFOTEH-JAHORINA, pp 1–6
38. Rathod J, Gupta A, Patel D (2020) using blockchain technology for continuing medical education credits system. In: 2020 seventh international conference on software defined systems (SDS), pp 214–9
39. Pradesh A, Council M, Of D, Services H, Guidelines for conducting cme programme & accreditation of cme credit hours framed by the sub committee on cme arunachal pradesh medical council. Directorate of health services complex, 2246708(161)

Blockchain in Education: Linking Competency Assessment with Credentialing

10

Travis P. Sharkey-Toppen, Timothy C. Hoffman, Kendra McCamey, and David P. Bahner

> *Schools in the future will be judged less because of the credentials that they bestow, and more because of the experiences that they offer.*
>
> –Roger Schank

Abstract

Blockchain is a distributed ledger where "write once, never erase" is the mantra for this digital record keeping. Physician and practitioner credentialing is the arduous, often repetitive process of verifying medical school diplomas, residency completion, and successful board certification and continued education. From medical board licensing to obtaining hospital privileges, the process is time-consuming, expensive and frequently requires an unseemly amount of blind trust regarding performance competency. This process has grown as non-physician providers expanded scope of practice and telemedicine laws loosened. Point-of-care ultrasound is an example of a procedural skill that can be learned and practiced in medicine. To practice it well is an essential physician and practitioner skill that has historically demonstrated significant variation between operators with varied experiences from medical school, residency, and hospital use. Block chain technology offers a solution by providing a natural ledger for standardized reporting of these various documents of competency but also a record

T. P. Sharkey-Toppen · T. C. Hoffman · D. P. Bahner (✉)
Department of Emergency Medicine, The Ohio State University Wexner Medical Center, Columbus, OH, USA
e-mail: david.bahner@osumc.edu

K. McCamey
Division of Sports Medicine, Department of Family Medicine, The Ohio State University Wexner Medical Center, Columbus, OH, USA

© The Author(s), under exclusive license to Springer Nature Switzerland AG 2023
S. Stawicki (ed.), *Blockchain in Healthcare*, Integrated Science 10,
https://doi.org/10.1007/978-3-031-14591-9_10

of the quality of procedures performed, including ultrasound. It also provides a direct means for universal distribution of credentialing for each provider by simplifying the process, making it more efficient with a new level of integrity.

Keywords

Blockchain · Ultrasound · Competency assessment · Credentialing · Assessment · Learning theory · Deliberate practice

Introduction

Without a good understanding of the technology involved, many may hear the idea of blockchain and may not understand what it means. There has been significant media coverage of the success of blockchain implementation due to the cryptocurrency boom in 2017 [1]. This focus on crypto has since experienced an ebb and flow as a demonstration of one of the first successful practical applications of blockchain [2]. Blockchain and cryptocurrency are not synonymous, however, and only represent a narrow understanding of the technology. In fact, large-scale initiatives seek to make these forms of distributed ledgers accessible, reliable, and easily applicable to large-scale solutions for varying business models, such as the Hyperledger project [3]. The goal being to provide transactions that can be verified once and stored without fear of biased corruption or manipulation. With support of these open-source initiatives by many interested parties, blockchain technology is likely to continue to become a potential solution for transactions that require a high level of integrity as is often needed in the healthcare industry [3].

Given its integrity and transparency, blockchain is an attractive technology that may be applied to many healthcare challenges. For example, patient remote monitoring, pharmaceutical verification, and secure patient identification are just a few of the many areas where this blockchain digitization of information could improve real world current processes. In this chapter, we explore the application of blockchain as a tool to improve the integrity and efficiency of current credentialing of medical providers.

Credentialing and Privileging of Medical Practitioners

One of the most exciting ways that blockchain could interface with medicine and medical education would be to serve as a new way to document competency for credentialing medical providers that is both more reliable and efficient than current methods. In fact, there have been several decades of calls for improvement to the credentialing system to provide a unified standard and reduce redundancy as well as implement software solutions to manage the complex process across institutions [4]. The healthcare workforce looks different with levels of expertise throughout the hospital. Hospital privileging which is local is a surrogate for credentialing thus it has no specific standard between individual clinics or other hospital systems. As a result, the process is often tedious, disjointed, and inconsistent both for the provider as well as the system performing the credentialing process.

Medical school training accredits because of curricular knowledge and experiences medical students accomplish typically during a 4-year matriculation. Then during residency, these new graduates, medical doctors or doctors of osteopathy, enter into a specialty field such as internal medicine, general surgery, family medicine, emergency medicine, radiology, anesthesiology and many more within the American Board of Medical Specialty (ABMS) [5]. The training has been compared to and equal to between 10,000 and 40,000 h of training [6], deliberate practice and various knowledge assessments amidst patient encounters and care. Each specialty has a Residency Review Committee (RRC) that reports to the Accreditation Council for Graduate Medical Education (ACGME) and functions with the Joint Commission on Accreditation of Healthcare Organizations as it relates to federal standards and funding [7].

For example, upon completion of residency, an Emergency Medicine resident must meet minimum competency benchmarks established by their certifying board, the American Board of Emergency Medicine (ABEM) [8]. These standards ensure that the physician is competent to perform various skills including multiple procedures such as intubation, ultrasound, and central lines. The performance of these skills during residency is recorded in various ways across varying Graduate Medical Education (GME) accredited programs for resident physicians. Each specialty program has a certifying board with specific qualifications for completion of required procedures related to medical expertise in that specialty. Typically, the performance of a required procedure or skill is also self-reported by the resident and therefore can have or lack verification from a supervisor who can ensure it was performed correctly or met that minimum competency standard. This record of skills is later used as a form of proof that they have competency in these skills and is verified by an attesting program director. Program directors ensure programs employ the latest mastery of learning principles that are not the norm yet. In fact, case logs completed by an individual are the typical standard for recording this information. This bears to question what value is there in maintaining a record that gains its validity from the person attempting to prove their competency in a system. It is possible this documentation and requirement of procedural competency may vary for nurse and physician assistant practitioners as well. Furthermore, there is no guarantee of integrity of even the maintenance of this record as it may be easily manipulated as necessary with no ability to verify its validity. This method of self-reporting procedures also can result in an underestimation of actual procedure numbers. An active learner is typically more focused on the performing procedures than reporting completions, leaving many procedures unattributed to their record.

Procedural competency for other providers such as nurse practitioners, physician assistants, optometrists, or even sonographers are different than the training for a physician. A physician can be a provider, but not all providers are physicians. A practitioner is involved in the practice of medicine and functions as part of the healthcare team. However, the disjointed nature of some medical encounters and care plans is manifest with busy waiting rooms in ED's and overflowing ICU's. In regard to medical practice, a spectrum of people and positions exist that "practice" medicine. Many times, a patient's "doctor" is a nurse practitioner or other advanced practice provider that does not have the same length or depth of training as a physician. Now these same issues are present amidst a changed landscape. The COVID-19 pandemic for example will be a reflection point for all the disparities in our system that have further stressed a system that was already operating with these constraints [9, 10].

Once graduated, a physician or practitioner would have to provide their training record to their new employer, and possibly multiple hospital systems depending on where they work, to undergo the credentialing process at their new location [11]. These requirements may vary widely by each hospital system in order to verify competency for credentialing. There is no true industry standard yet or evidence-based standard except primary recommendations and letters of reference. This may require searching through multiple sources of files, e-mails, or other forms of records to provide what is often unverified documentation to demonstrate competency. This process is likely to repeat itself, but rarely the same way twice, throughout an individual's career further emphasizing the lack of consistency or even relevancy of how some of this credentialing is performed. This can be true even for doctors practicing within the same region having different requirements for the same procedures at different hospitals. Physicians that practice locum tenens or those participating in telemedicine may even see an increase in complexity to accommodate a wider variety of these hospital systems, each with a nuanced view of medical credentialing from state to state. What is their value as physicians with expert knowledge versus a mid-level advanced practitioner that knows the local area, doctors and practice patterns? When does opinion become more of an expert opinion? Opinions are not facts.

Now imagine that there is a better way to document and track this information. Imagine instead that a physician can easily document their performance of a specific procedure and have it verified by a supervisor. This witness would provide verification of their competency in performance of a given task. Further, this verification is then stored in a trusted record that is standardized, easily read and shared, but difficult if not impossible to falsely manipulate. From a practical view, this would streamline the credentialing process. Each credentialing body would merely query the record for a skill that is being requested by the provider to verify demonstrated competency.

This system would also be beneficial to the learning environment. Attending physicians could quickly and discreetly check the credentials of a resident physician or other mid-level provider to ensure her or his qualifications prior to performing a given procedure. This too provides an advantage, replacing the current system where a resident may be tempted to overstate her or his proficiency at a given procedure just to get the opportunity to perform it. Instead, the attending would be able to check their record of procedures and teach accordingly.

Blockchain has the potential to provide the above stated reality. It would provide a secure record that could be universally shared between institutions who require credentialing or supervised training to maintain verification of their competency to perform their job. Making this available direct to consumer (patient) before each procedure is another reality depending on how the blockchain is created and maintained. Blockchain is a technology. Strategic directions in the delivery of healthcare are afforded to the leaders and innovators inside and outside the healthcare system.

Current Credentialing Process

One example of the difficulty with the current medical credentialing process is shown with the rapid growth of point-of-care ultrasound (POCUS) and the need to credential providers to utilize this complex imaging procedure. Ultrasound has been called operator dependent meaning the skill was dependent on the operator. It was hard to learn and perform and still is to a degree. The use of POCUS in healthcare has rapidly grown and a requisite training infrastructure in emergency and critical care has outpaced the use of POCUS in primary or basic surgical/medical care. As the cost of entry continues to lower with the development of handheld ultrasound devices, it continues to become a more accessible but powerful tool in trained hands to improve rapid diagnosis and procedural guidance in a variety of medical conditions. However, the performance of those who use ultrasound could be "operator dependent", meaning it is up to the training of each individual operator that determines the skill and competency of the completed ultrasound procedure. The key to its success comes from the incredible training efforts of the pioneers, who conceptualized this novel skill set and implemented it first in specific individual programs and then more broadly into the individual specialty practices [12–18]. The technology has diffused even further with wider adoption by mid-level advanced practice providers. Yet the practice of medicine involves over 25 medical specialty boards and the performance of POCUS by members of each specialty varies across the fields and disciplines of medicine. Individual motivation, accessibility of the new technology, organizational infrastructure of the medical workplace and imaging logistics all impact the quality and quantity of POCUS in a variety of professional medical settings that exist.

The goal of medical credentialing is to show that a healthcare provider has had adequate training and has proven competency to practice in a certain field or to perform a certain procedure. Ultrasound is not new and multiple specialties have varying levels of experience with integrating ultrasound into their workflow such as radiology, cardiology, obstetrics/gynecology, emergency medicine, and critical care medicine [12, 13, 16–18]. Comprehensive exams typically are obtained by sonographers and interpreted by imaging specialists while point-of-care ultrasound (POCUS) exams are usually done by the clinician sonologist. This term and many others describe the users who practice POCUS. These specialty residency and even fellowship programs have varying experience with formal training in the acquisition and interpretation of ultrasound for the varying applications relevant to that specialty (e.g. vascular, musculoskeletal ultrasound). The more formalized this education is, the easier it is to recognize what level of competency is to be expected for the credentialing process. However, even if these minimum competency standards are met, gathering the information needed for initial credentialing as well as the maintenance of that competency over time is both time consuming but also with varying levels of validity. For example, one institution may require direct review of a certain number of acquired images and their interpretation by a resident physician in order to verify competency, while another program may only rely on self-reporting of ultrasounds being performed on shift for verification in a log. Likewise, reporting of this competency to a credentialing body may vary from a self-reported list of performed ultrasounds to verification from a third party such as the ultrasound director where they trained, or a residency program director.

Once completed, it is the responsibility of credentialing committee in individual networks to authenticate the skills, letters of recommendations, certifications, licensure and other forms of verification in order to allow a physician or provider to practice in that single network. It is often described as slow, painful, redundant and sometimes felt to be arbitrary at times. Once a provider has been credentialed, they need to show that they have maintained their skill and competency with periodic review of credentialing. The cadence of this maintenance of certification has been debated among specialty groups. Documenting and showing the continued competency can be difficult. In fact, with the growing number of providers as well as the easier access to technology such as ultrasound, it becomes impractical to dedicate human work hours to the rigor that may be required to verify a provider's maintenance of skills over time with the same level of scrutiny that was given to initial credentialing. This is true of all skills.

To further complicate the situation, there are no accepted standards across institutions and their multitude of specialties regarding the requirements for initial or continued competency verification for skills such as ultrasound. If a provider leaves one institution to join another or practices at multiple institutions at once, the credentialing process is likely to be done independently at each institution. This can be both frustrating for providers and can result in a significant delay in becoming credentialed. The process can be months to 6 months in order to verify references, letters, and curriculum vitae. It is also a time-consuming and expensive venture for the institutions themselves [19].

Technological Advantages and Challenges of Blockchain

When someone hears of blockchain, the term is typically associated with cryptocurrency. This is only one single example of what can be achieved using this technology. Blockchain is the technology that allows transparency and open-source ledgering to track a set of information. The integrity and security of the data stored in blockchain are its strengths and since its digital infrastructure knows no borders its ubiquity for a global citizenry is endless. Blockchain is not restrictive to financial applications and has a much broader applicability especially in healthcare [20–24].

Fundamentally, blockchain is a form of database [25]. Traditional databases have a table structure with each column of the table representing some value that we wish to store in a record and each row representing a single record [26]. In its simplest form, these tables are represented by spreadsheets where someone is free to manipulate each cell within the table as necessary. This form of database prioritizes the ease of access of information. It often has columns reserved to provide some form of timestamp that keeps track of when the record was created, or possibly when it was last updated. There are also ways to manipulate more complex databases to keep a record of these changes, but this is not intuitive nor efficient in these forms of databases.

Blockchain, however, prioritizes true chronological record keeping [25]. Each block in a chain can represent a record or set of records that was entered into the database at some point in time. When the block is finalized, it is concatenated to the chain, thus naturally creating a timeline of records or what is commonly referred to as a transaction in this model. If applied to credentialing, one may track each verified course, scan, prior credentialing, or other pertinent documentation as part of a record or transaction. These transactions would then persist no matter what status changes may happen in the future, and the blockchain itself becomes a timeline of every event that was ever recorded since it was initiated.

For example, assume a provider fails to obtain credentialing or has their credentialing revoked, but later gets re-credentialed. In the case of a traditional database, it may only keep track of the current snapshot of this record and show that the provider is currently credentialed at a particular institution. In the case of blockchain, these transitions in status would be able to be seen or queried by credentialing bodies in the future. Traditional databases can be structured to maintain historical data, but this is typically more cumbersome and inefficient by comparison [26]. Layers of information can become transparent when chronologically tracked along the chain.

One might ask at this point, "what stops a person from manipulating older blocks to change their transactions?" Could a provider who has had his privileges revoked, hack the blockchain and change the credentialing record? As blocks are added to a chain, multiple events will occur and how this process works can vary depending on how the blockchain was designed and who is maintaining the integrity of the blockchain. The first thing to understand, is that each block is dependent on the data that was added before it in how the data is encoded into the block. Each block contains its own "hash" that is a calculation that is done using the current data in the block as well as the hash of the block that it is attached to in the chain [27]. If someone was to maliciously change information to a past event, it would then corrupt all data that comes afterwards. This can be easily identified and the data on that blockchain would then not be trusted. In order to circumvent this and maliciously manipulate a chain, one must update the data for every subsequent block in order to make the chain valid again.

This should lead to the next question, "how difficult would it be to update every block in order to manipulate a single transaction?" In order to add transactions in a block and the block then be added to a chain, computationally expensive work must be performed that is commonly referred to as proof of work. These calculations typically require expensive hardware, time, and high-energy costs in order to process, which de-incentivizes someone from using this as a way to manipulate the system. In common implementations, this proof-of-work is regulated to maintain a given level of difficulty that is scalable [28]. It is therefore conceivable for someone to attempt to manipulate a chain, but unlikely to be rewarding due to its high cost.

Traditional transactions take place at the local level, or with the framework of state, national or international boundaries. Furthermore, blockchain can be made more secure by decentralizing the database itself [25]. This may seem counterintuitive to previous calls for making a centralized credentialing system, which is still possible even with a decentralized database. It may be good to consider this a unified decentralized database in order to avoid confusion. Traditional databases are usually stored by a single entity that becomes an authority over that data. Banking is probably the easiest analogy to consider when it comes to understanding this concept. An individual can go to a bank, either digitally or physically, and deposit money that the bank stores for them. Now, banks do not physically take the money given to it and keep it in a safe and then return those exact same bills physically to that individual when requested. Rather, a record is kept of that transaction as well as a summary of the current state or balance of that individual's account. When the individual needs the money back, they make a request from the bank who deducts the amount from their current balance. In this example, the bank is responsible for record keeping and becomes the authority over how much money that individual has stored there. Of course, this gives the bank a significant amount of power over the individual as an authority over their money. It may become difficult for the customer to dispute any discrepancies. There are accountability measures in place in the traditional system, but it still puts significant faith in the bank itself to maintain credible records.

Now contrast the model of a traditional bank to a blockchain model of banking or cryptocurrency. Blockchain has already been discussed as a database that is secure with easily verifiable data [2]. Blockchain can also live on multiple computers that all have the same verification strategy and therefore should be stored with identical information, and thus a unified dataset. If a person wants to verify the integrity of the data from any one source, one can simply query all the available computers that maintain this blockchain to verify that the information is the same. If the record being verified differs from the majority of the other instances of the blockchain, it is considered corrupt and therefore would be considered an invalid or untrusted source. This decentralized database was the impetus for the use of blockchain as a way to maintain what is known as cryptocurrency because it takes the authority away from a central body or bank and gives it to anyone wishing to participate in the maintenance of the blockchain. Although a single entity may earn trust over time, it is hard to argue that it is easier to trust a large number of sources with the same information. In the case of credentialing, it may be prudent to house these systems within the various healthcare systems that perform credentialing and shared as a unified network with an accepted standard.

There are some limitations that should be considered in the implementation of a system that relies on blockchain. Probably the most daunting of these is the cost of adding information to a blockchain. As was discussed, it is computationally expensive to add a block to the chain. Although there are many providers that could eventually see their credentialing information placed on a blockchain, the frequency and volume of these types of transactions is far fewer than what would be seen in the more common usage of blockchain as a form of cryptocurrency. Each transaction would serve as a representation of significant information related to a provider's training and competency, such as completing a board examination, obtaining licensure, or performing a supervised procedure. Each of these take time and significant effort to achieve and are therefore rare compared to the frequency of transactions in a cryptocurrency model. As such, it is safe to infer that since the cryptocurrency model has been demonstrated to be achievable that a much less demanding implementation would also be obtainable. Another more adept comparison would be to consider the cost of third-party verification of skills. The costs associated with a blockchain implementation would then be offset by the savings in requiring less human time spent dedicated to credentialing and maintenance of records. The energy output of mining the blockchain is another consideration as well as its disruption of current systems of providing service.

Blockchain introduces many advantages as well as disadvantages compared to our current forms of record keeping. Verification of competency is reduced to querying the blockchain for required existing credentials that occurred at some transaction along the chain. It no longer relies on documentation or reproduction of information that is reliant on a single entity or perhaps person to provide. This also eliminates the need for third-party verification if it is stored in a decentralized manner that is made widely available for audit. Furthermore, this decentralized schema makes it difficult to manipulate for malicious purposes (see Table 10.1).

Table 10.1 Comparison of blockchain to traditional databases

Blockchain	Traditional database
Complete history	Snapshot of the Current State
Difficult to manipulate existing records	Easy to manipulate existing Records
Typically stored as a decentralized database	Typically stored as a centralized database
Relatively expensive to add a new record or block to the chain	Relatively inexpensive to add a new record to the database

A Changing Landscape

With the introduction and adoption of electronic medical record systems quickly phasing out the need for paper charting, medicine has already started down the inevitable pathway to a digitally managed system. Currently whether you pick up your medications at a pharmacy, have them delivered by drone, examine your own "chart" online, or wear an electronic fitness device; our lives are becoming digitized. The traditional healthcare encounter has changed but whether digital or in person: what is the "value" of expert opinion? What is the value of opinion? How much training distinguishes opinion from expert opinion? In medicine, this process is known as credentialing and was used as the final step to ensure patients were being treated by doctors skilled and experienced to perform diagnostics and therapeutics. As other practitioners became involved in the practice of medicine from nurses and nurse practitioners to physician assistants and optometrists have expanded scope and all of this increased with telemedicine. The value of a healthcare visit is based on the knowledge, experience, and care provided by physicians and practitioners of healthcare during the pandemic and afterward. The qualifications matter and so does experience, yet the virtual methods were new to us all in 2020, and some are adapting better than others. There will be a new normal and sometimes it takes decades to settle some things before the next major stressor, or maybe sooner.

As the world continues to understand the COVID-19 pandemic, the shift to more digitally supported life has become even more apparent in all of society. Authentication, authorization, and verification of data transfer has become a ubiquitous part of daily life in almost every business realm with medicine being central to the health of us all. Authentic facilities, authorized providers of new technology, verified practitioners currently exist and current credentialing although cumbersome, functions and works. But the pandemic put new stresses on this system. As providers work across state lines or volunteer in other areas of need, credentialing delays prevent flexibility. Plus, state laws for independent practice of advanced practice providers confounds practice autonomy as belies the lack of one national standard.

Further, medicine in the United States has been pushed to expand access to medicine in multiple ways since the introduction of the Affordable Care Act of 2010 [29]. This law, among other considerations, saw expanded funding for mid-level providers to increase their support, scope-of-practice, and even minimize their requirements to begin practice in clinical medicine. This has expanded with telemedicine and administrators looking at all employees as providers, and many times, just trying to staff their service lines. The requirements of these providers are different, and in fact all providers from prehospital care with emergency medical technicians, paramedics, mid-level providers such as nurse practitioners and physician assistants as well as the physicians they all practice under varies widely in their skills and the credentialing required to give them the privilege to practice medicine. There is an organization, a process, and some similarities but all vary and are unique to their individual specialty and field of study. Expanding the scope of differently trained providers than physicians is an administrative decision and the blockchain can handle varying levels of verification and authorization of skills, whichever strategic direction an organization wants to take. More advanced practice providers are many times seen as a pathway to alleviate the burden of too few providers for an ever-growing population demand. However, when their autonomy runs aground of expert medical opinion for numbers of hours trained and medical ability, there is a difference in their levels of expertise and competency compared to a physician counterpart. It is in the raw numbers and hours of coursework, patient hours, academic rigor between medical school programs and other disciplines that bears the cost for this expertise. There are many bottlenecks before, during, and even after initial training in order to ensure all providers are well trained and ready for the challenges ahead and credentialing is often seen as the last hurdle in order to get these providers into the workforce and start caring for patients.

As the number of providers continues to increase throughout medicine, the demand for high-quality care is still a basic expectation which means there cannot be a compromise in the qualifications of those practitioners seeking to provide care. Further, these qualifications change over time, both as the practice of medicine changes, but also the skills of any provider dependent on the environment in which they practice and their own initiative to challenge themselves and knowledge obtained through continued practice and education. As such, competency is not a static target, but rather a fluid goal that requires a lifetime of continued lifelong learning, maintenance of skills, and direct-patient care experience. Knowledge plus experience equals layers of expertise. These concrete items technically can be collected and linked to a person's authentic record of professional ability. Agreeing on a format and implementation logistics are institutional system decisions, yet the technology exists for current deployment. Will future credentialing of procedures be logged on blockchain? However, it is an impractical expectation to report and repeatedly verify each of the experiences that prove competency through modern credentialing practices. Balancing privacy, security, and logging cases for quality assurance or continued medical education (CME) are essential yet not currently prioritized so that practitioners are primed to maximize their potential from lifelong learning. If expertise grows over time, do more senior providers get recognized for longevity, expertise or wisdom? Does it matter for patients? The blockchain disruption may be an opportunity to tackle the nuance of skill and expertise. What separates opinion from expert opinion? This demands a significant change. In order to provide a reliable system to overcome the technical and strategic components of this credentialing conundrum there needs to be the vision to determine inclusive, equitable, accountable solutions to these challenges in the construct of a more blockchain centric healthcare system.

The Vision

As with the existing credentialing system, the goal is to get verified results of past experiences that demonstrate competency of a given provider in order to safely allow for privileges in a given healthcare system. Figure 10.1 demonstrates the general flow of this information from completion of tests of competency (e.g., proctored or quality reviewed procedure such as an ultrasound acquisition and interpretation, reporting of examination scores, certificates of completion such as Advanced Cardiac Life Support [ACLS], Advanced Trauma Life Support [ATLS]) to requests for confirmation of skills by healthcare systems as privileges are being granted or reviewed for a new or existing provider.

Providers demonstrate their competency through typical methods, including board examinations, certifications, as well as demonstration of skills in supervised experiences such as simulations or real-life demonstration of skills such as ultrasound. Certifying bodies, including supervisors witnessing this competency, verify

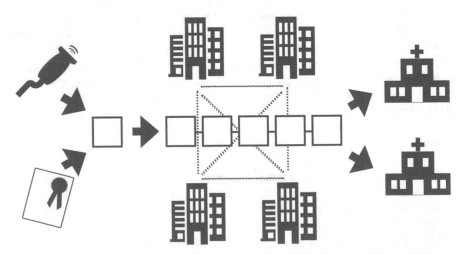

Fig. 10.1 The flow of verification of competency from real-time completion that is added to a block. This block gets submitted to the blockchain, which is decentralized on a distributed ledger between participating institutions. Healthcare systems can then query this database for the desired information about a provider in order to streamline their credentialing process

the completion along with any quality scores such as board scores, procedure outcomes, image acquisition quality, and other relevant information. These verified results get added to a block that is submitted to the credentialing blockchain. This new block is verified and added to the chain at participating institutions. These participating institutions should include but not necessarily be limited to training programs (e.g., residency and fellowship programs), certifying bodies (e.g., National Board of Medical Examiners, American Board of Emergency Medicine, American Heart Association), and healthcare systems. As a decentralized system, no single institution would therefore be seen as a sole authority of this process which would maintain a fair representation of all providers history. As shared consumers of this information, they would also contribute to the shared cost of maintaining this system. When it comes time to credential a new provider or to ensure maintenance of skills, a healthcare system simply queries the blockchain for necessary transactions to confirm competency. This could be done by querying a specific piece of information such as ACLS certification but could also be accomplished by requesting a query on a provider's entire dossier for the credentialing committee to review.

It is important to recognize that except for participation in completing a competency assessment, a provider is removed from this process, alleviating the laborious task of collecting and reporting of this information for the provider which as has been discussed comes with many disadvantages beyond the inconvenience of the task. Further, although this system is designed to accomplish credentialing for privileges of providers, it could also be used for establishing current completions as part of a training program, with the end consumer being the training program rather than the healthcare system they may also serve.

Conclusion

Blockchain as it has been described may be a solution that could provide a one-time verification of competency in a skill, present and accessible to any healthcare system as it considers privileges of a physician or provider to practice medicine. It can be seen as a trusted source material that could be shared between institutions of medicine in order to expedite the process of verification of skills. This already could decrease the inefficiency of manual transfer of various forms of verification that exist today. Furthermore, this would present a challenge to formulate a standard for reporting to maintain consistency that would be also transparent to all parties with access to the ledger. In fact, it may be reasonable to speculate with standardization and readily accessible information on such a ledger that this process could become at least in part automated. A physician or practitioner requests privileges in a given healthcare setting with privileges to perform specific procedures or interventions in the support of that population. A tailored software program could then verify against the ledger that this provider has met the standards for competency based on the experiences or transactions that have previously been verified and stored on this digital timeline. As a physician or practitioner continues through practice, it can continue to verify expectations for continued education and practical experiences that would also be stored on the same ledger. This process could then continue throughout the person's career, minimizing interruptions in practice but also identifying professionals whose skills may have dissipated due to lack of continued experience or education to maintain competency. In fact, clarifying reputation, and authenticating expertise using blockchain would greatly strengthen the reliability of all physicians, practitioners, and providers within the practice of medicine for the good of patients and beyond.

References

1. Griffin JM, Shams A (2019) Is bitcoin really un-tethered? https://papers.ssrn.com/abstract=3195066. https://doi.org/10.2139/ssrn.3195066
2. Nakamoto S (2008) Bitcoin: a peer-to-peer electronic cash system
3. Hyperledger–open source blockchain technologies. https://www.hyperledger.org/
4. Cole JW (1998) Physician credentialing. A centralized verification system. Phys Exec 24:52–55
5. About ABMS. American board of medical specialties. https://www.abms.org/about-abms/
6. Brown B The deceptive income of physicians. http://benbrownmd.wordpress.com/.
7. Institutional application and requirements. https://www.acgme.org/designated-institutional-officials/institutional-review-committee/institutional-application-and-requirements/
8. About ABEM. https://www.abem.org/public/about-abem
9. CDC (2020) Health equity considerations and racial and ethnic mintority groups. Centers for Disease Control and Prevention. https://www.cdc.gov/coronavirus/2019-ncov/community/health-equity/race-ethnicity.html
10. Leung TI, Biskup E, DeWitt D (2020) Facilitating credentialing and engagement of international physician-migrants during the COVID-19 crisis and beyond. Rural Remote Health 20:6027
11. Hittle K (2010) Understanding certification, licensure, and credentialing: a guide for the new nurse practitioner. J Pediatr Health Care 24:203–206
12. Heller MB et al (2002) Residency training in emergency ultrasound: fulfilling the mandate. Acad Emerg Med Off J Soc Acad Emerg Med 9:835–839
13. Andruszkiewicz P, Sobczyk D (2013) Ultrasound in critical care. Anaesthesiol Intensive Ther 45:177–181
14. Bornemann P, Barreto T (2018) Point-of-care ultrasonography in family medicine. Am Fam Phys 98:200–202
15. Soni NJ et al (2019) Point-of-care ultrasound for hospitalists: a position statement of the society of hospital medicine. J Hosp Med. https://doi.org/10.12788/jhm.3079
16. Almufleh A, Di Santo P, Marbach JA (2019) Training cardiology fellows in focused cardiac ultrasound. J Am Coll Cardiol 73:1097–1100
17. Alrahmani L, Codsi E, Borowski KS (2018) The current state of ultrasound training in obstetrics and gynecology residency programs. J Ultrasound Med Off J Am Inst Ultrasound Med 37:2201–2207
18. Suarez-Weiss KE, Yang H, Beland MD (2020) Reclaiming hands-on ultrasound for radiology with a simulation-based ultrasound curriculum for radiology residents. Ultrasound Q 36:268–274
19. O'Kane M (2002) Verify, but please, only once. Physician credentialing is important, but too many are doing too much of it. Mod Healthc 32:17

20. Abdullah S, Rothenberg S, Siegel E, Kim W (2020) School of block-review of blockchain for the radiologists. Acad Radiol 27:47–57
21. Justinia T (2019) Blockchain technologies: opportunities for solving real-world problems in healthcare and biomedical sciences. Acta Inform Medica AIM J Soc Med Inform Bosnia Herzeg Cas Drustva Za Med Inform BiH 27:284–291
22. Kamel Boulos MN, Wilson JT, Clauson KA (2018) Geospatial blockchain: promises, challenges, and scenarios in health and healthcare. Int J Health Geogr 17:25
23. Mackey TK et al (2019) 'Fit-for-purpose?'-challenges and opportunities for applications of blockchain technology in the future of healthcare. BMC Med 17:68
24. Mackey TK, Miyachi K, Fung D, Qian S, Short J (2020) Combating health care fraud and abuse: conceptualization and prototyping study of a blockchain antifraud framework. J Med Internet Res 22:e18623
25. Ethereum Whitepaper. ethereum.org. https://ethereum.org
26. Halpin T, Morgan T (2010) Information modeling and relational databases. Morgan Kaufmann
27. Lamport L (1981) Password authentication with insecure communication. Commun ACM 24:770–772
28. Developer Guides—Bitcoin. https://developer.bitcoin.org/devguide/
29. McIntyre A, Song Z (2019) The US affordable care act: reflections and directions at the close of a decade. PLoS Med 16:e1002752

Optimizing Blockchain Technology in Academic Medicine

11

Kathryn C. Kelley and Anthony P. Allsbrook

> *Medical education does not exist to provide students with a way of making a living, but to ensure the health of the community.*
>
> –Rudolf Virchow

Abstract

Academic medicine is certainly an area in which blockchain technology could add efficiency, simplicity, and security for learners, educational institutions, and even potential employers. A career in Medicine fundamentally requires a lifelong commitment of continuing education, learning and developing new skillsets, and scholarship. This chapter serves to highlight specific instances in which blockchain ledger could be applied to areas in academic medicine, including the maintenance of academic records, tracking of academic achievement and scholarly work, and the forum for exchange secure information (i.e. medical board testing, employment contracts). By providing specific instances where blockchain could be potentially be valuable to medical education, this chapter may serve as inspiration for further applications of blockchain into the educational landscape.

Keywords

Blockchain · Tokenization · Academic medicine · Medical education · Academic records · Cryptocurrency

K. C. Kelley (✉) · A. P. Allsbrook
St. Luke's University Health Network, 801 Ostrum St., Bethlehem, PA, USA
e-mail: Kathryn.kelley@sluhn.org

A. P. Allsbrook
e-mail: Anthony.Allsbrook@sluhn.org

Introduction

Blockchain technology is gaining increased awareness as a revolutionary format for the secure storage of transactions and the exchanges of ideas amongst peers. Blockchain has numerous applications in Healthcare and Medicine, but of particular interest is its potential role in Medical Education. Physicians accrue a considerable amount of knowledge, skills, and accolades during their careers, with no simple way to validate and authenticate these career milestones [1]. Blockchain enters as a means to simplify and track records and credentials. The guiding principles of blockchain are the following: transparency, efficiency, and anonymity; the technology serves as an "electronic ledger," where "blocks" represent a series of transactions. "Blocks" are then encrypted with an algorithm, with a series of blocks denoting a "blockchain." A blockchain is then able to be distributed widely across entire networks of peers, with the ability for all who have ownership to add new blocks [2]. Integrity is maintained in the chain by ensuring that no block can be individually modified without creating disruption of the entire chain [2]. With such a strong system of data integrity, one can easily view how blockchain could become an asset in the areas of Medical Education where data breaches and/or maintenance of verifiable information are of utmost concern, including: tracking accurate academic records and grading for students, "tokenization" of academic awards, achievements, and accolades, and secure systems in which licensing, contracts, and testing can be conducted. In its inherent form, blockchain is certainly able to become a reliable format for storing and authenticating individual academic records [2] (see Fig. 11.1).

Fig. 11.1 Potential Areas for Utilization of Blockchain Technology in Academic Medicine

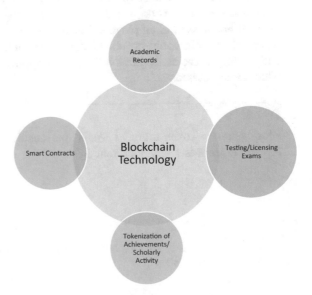

Using Blockchain for Academic Records

Blockchain technology can potentially serve as a cheaper and more reliable substitute to the current standard of the paper official transcripts [3]. The antiquated official transcript continues to play an important role in evaluating qualifications of prospective students or employers. The document, which is owned and managed by specific universities or institutions, provides a transcript that contains information such as courses completed, grades, and credits received. There are obvious issues with this antiquated system. Blockchain technology can make this process faster, safer, and more reliable [3]. To illustrate an example, in 2017, the Massachusetts Institute of Technology (MIT) developed a blockchain-based app, "Digital Diplomas," in 2017 to allow students to share "tamper-proof digital versions" of their degrees with potential employers or other institutions [4, 5]. Additionally, in 2016, the Sony Corporation, via its initiative Sony Global Education, publicized their plans to "build a blockchain for the 'open and secure sharing of academic proficiency and progress records'" [6].

In the current educational system, a student requests an official transcript from the specific institution for a fee and the transcript is mailed to its intended destination. Since each transcript is maintained at the individual institution, the student must rely on administration to retrieve and send off their records. This process becomes even more tedious for students who attend multiple institutions throughout their educational journey [3]. This is a common occurrence as the National Student Clearinghouse in 2018 showed that approximately 37% of students will transfer prior to obtaining a degree [7]. Sharples (2016) argues that an obvious clinical use of blockchain is to store records of achievement and credit. This data can be added to the blockchain by the awarding institution which the student would be able to access and share. This provides a consistent public record in one decentralized place that is protected from changes in the institution or potential loss of records [8].

Not only is this process difficult for the applicant it is tedious and taxing to the evaluating authority as they must confirm validity from each institution. Chen et al. [9] proposes that blockchain technology has the potential to reduce degree fraud by allowing blockchain to grant and manage a student's degree and transcript [9]. Since data matched with each student is validated and checked by miners all over, fraud will be significantly reduced [9]. Swamy and Parmar [10] also discuss the major drawbacks of the current practice in terms of obtaining an official transcript, highlighting the ease with which transcripts can be tampered, but also noting it can be difficult to detect these illegitimate alterations [10]. Chen et al. were able to propose an inexpensive academic transcript system using blockchain technology that provides both security and transparency while reducing cost [10].

One of the most obvious uses of blockchain technology in academics is within the realm of academic records. The current standard of distributing academic records is outdated and leads to a time-consuming process that is difficult on both the student and evaluating institution. Blockchain technology provides an affordable system that safely protects a student's records all while improving storage, transferability, and reliability.

Tokenization of Academic Achievements

The idea of "tokenization" in regards to blockchain technology refers to the formatting of a nondigital achievement or asset into a blockchain-based unit, or "token" [2]. Items that can be "tokenized" include any academic awards, faculty promotions, or research citations. For example, Kosmarski [11] suggests that "one could receive tokens if their research results are validated independently by others, or used in their future work, thus serving as an economic equivalent of citation" [11]. By tokenizing these scholastic and career achievements, the process of student/faculty advancement, evaluation of performance, and the hiring process become overall simpler. As medical education, in particular, is a process of "lifelong learning," tokens on a blockchain ledger could continue to grow over an individual's career, "archiving every conference attended, every article written, and rates of successful treatment for every patient encountered or procedure performed" [5].

With these concepts in mind, Turkanović et al. of Slovenia devised a blockchain-focused higher education credit platform titled "EduCTX," which is based on the European Credit Transfer and Accumulation System (ECTS) [12]. EduCTX employs blockchain technology to create a higher education credit and grading system. Students can view their completed courses in a single view, and universities, thus, can access all of this data in real time [12]. One of the motivations for devising EduCTX was simplifying the hiring process for recent university graduates; when graduates went to apply for job positions, sometimes in a different country than their country of education, they had difficulty validating their academic degrees due to lack of standardization, disorganization, or inaccessibility [12]. Students occasionally even had to go through a "nostrification process," including translating and converting/matching their official documentation and coursework to the language and curriculum of the hiring institution [12]. The EduCTX Platform suggests using "ECTX tokens" as a form of academic credit, allowing a peer-to-peer network to be utilized among students, hiring organizations, and institutions of higher education. Each student would maintain a "EduCTX blockchain wallet," and obtain tokens in the corresponding value of credits for their completed courses, thus being able to validate their academic record by simply presenting their blockchain address to an academic institution or potential employer [12].

Mohan [13] also argues that blockchain technology and tokenization can aid in combatting the growing problem of academic misconduct [13]. A 2009 meta-analysis found that on average, 2% of scientists "admitted to having fabricated, falsified, or modified data, while 14% knew colleagues who had done so … up to 33% admitted to some form of other 'questionable research practice,' and 72% expressed awareness of colleagues engaging in such practices" [13, 14]. Blockchain tcchnology, akin to anti-plagiarism software, can chiefly serve as a method to increase "probability of detection" [13, 15]. Scholars and researchers can be rewarded with tokens for policing or "refereeing" literature and detecting plagiarism or misconduct [13]. Thus, the integrity of the research community is reinforced through this unique application of technology.

While tokenization of academic achievements, degrees, citations, and various other entities demonstrates clear value of blockchain technology in the area of Medical Education, it is important to also note blockchain's utility in creating a secure space for transactions such as testing, obtaining/renewing medical licenses, and contracts for potential training or job positions.

Creating a Secure Space for Academic Transactions

The concept of "blockchain-based smart contracts" has been well-documented and posed as a safe method for data-protected transactions [16]. Via the utilization of advanced techniques of encryption, blockchain-based secure contracts have the potential to "provide a backbone for immutable paper-free employment (e.g. contracts) and IP-related (e.g. licensing and royalty payment) agreements" [2, 16]. Similar to conventional contracts, blockchain-based contracts define the terms of agreement, but are automatically processed once the necessary data requirements are met [4]. Thus, the agreements are enacted without the need for any mediator and are rendered both traceable and unalterable [4]. For example, in 2018, the world's first blockchain university was developed on the basis of smart contracts, Woolf University [4]. An online-based institution formed by scholars at Oxford University (UK), Woolf University uses blockchain smart contracts to record attendance, regulate payments, and track academic success [4]. Woolf University students select "modules" on an app to earn credits for undergraduate degrees, and "Woolf tokens" are used for fees [4]. Without the need to hire additional staff and administrators to act as "mediators" between students and instructors, Woolf thus strives to have lower course fees and higher pay for instructors [4].

The applications for blockchain-based smart contracts in academic medicine are severalfold. These secure contracts could potentially become the basis of State Board licensing for Physicians, Nurses, and other allied healthcare professionals, simplifying the process of verification and renewal of these credentials. Additionally, smart contracts could be used for hiring of medical professionals and academic staff by hospitals and university-based health systems, easily and quickly authenticating an applicant's qualifications, academic record, achievements, test scores, and even potentially performing criminal background checks. In the event that records are misplaced or lost (i.e. physicians who have relocated, are seeking asylum, or do not have access to their primary institutions of education), a blockchain record would be immediately available [1]. Naqvi and Hussain provide such an example where a physician from Syria relocates to the UK: the Syrian physician receives his diploma on a blockchain and owns the 'private keys' to his blockchain account [1]. The UK Medical Council is able to use the 'hash,' or unique digital stamp, on his blockchain account, to independently verify his credentials, without needing to contact his institution of education in Syria and easing the hiring process [1].

Another important area to which these secure systems could be applied is academic testing, particularly the high-stakes instances of board testing or licensing exams. For instance, in July 2020, during the attempted virtual administration of the American Board of Surgery (ABS) Qualifying Exam, the online system crashed, with concerns for potential privacy concerns and security breaches via a third-party proctoring system [17]. Testing candidates were required to provide "control of their computers, cameras, and phones, along with facial scans, passports, and drivers licenses" in order to test, leaving candidates in a vulnerable position once the testing system failed and forcing the ABS to launch a security investigation, "demanding the third party system delete all candidates' personal information and to provide evidence that they [had] done so" [17, 18]. Utilization of a secure, blockchain-based system for online testing may be extremely valuable in the future to prevent these potential security breaches from occurring during pivotal examinations.

Discussion

Evidence of blockchain-based technology's potential utility in academic medicine continues to grow. In general, the use of blockchain is following a "fairly typical pattern of adoption," with the numerous creations of cryptocurrencies/ blockchain apps worldwide in a competitive fashion [19]. Therefore, the time is nearing where practical blockchain-based solutions can be implemented into clinical and academic medicine [19]. The critical, rate-limiting step to application and use will be buy-in from academic institutions,

Implementation of blockchain into the medical education infrastructure will certainly require collaboration among academic institutions and learners [1]. Academic institutions will be required to adapt and transition to blockchain methods of record keeping, which may prove to be a time-consuming process for some. However, if blockchain offers a more secure, easily accessible method of storing this information, institutions may be persuaded in adopting the technology in a more expeditious fashion. Additionally, if potential employers are seeking information from students in a blockchain format, this may also be a guiding force for institutions to provide this beneficial tool to their learners.

Blockchain technology is not without its disadvantages; among the ones identified include potential financial issues. The possible concern has been posed that electricity and implementation costs could offset any savings incurred by hiring less staff or administrators or time management gains via more efficient documentation systems [1]. This chapter serves to highlight just a few prospective uses of blockchain technology to advance medical education in the areas of record keeping, tokenization of achievements, and secure means of testing/licensing/exchanges of contracts and to perhaps inspire new innovations and applications of blockchain to revolutionize the structure of academic medicine.

Conclusion

Although implementation will require a transition period and widespread adoption, there is significant evidence that Academic Medicine can certainly benefit from utilization of blockchain technology. By providing an avenue for efficient, secure storage of sensitive information, such as academic records, scholarly activity, licensing testing results, and other components of an academic profile, those within the Medical Education process can be offered a simplistic, protected, verifiable format for organizing their achievements. There is currently a paucity of literature with regard to function of blockchain-based applications in healthcare and medicine, and much additional research is warranted before broad spectrum implementation.

References

1. Naqvi N, Hussain M (2018) Medical education on the blockchain. J Br Blockchain Assoc 1
2. Stawicki S, Firstenberg M, Papadimos T (2018) What's new in academic medicine? Blockchain technology in health-care: bigger, better, fairer, faster, and leaner. Int J Acad Med 4(1):1–11
3. Maaghul R (2019) Blockchain credential for academia. https://medium.com/blockchain-and-the-distributed-workforce/blockchain-credentials-for-academia-9d4e05cedbeb
4. Williams P (2019) Does competency-based education with blockchain signal a new mission for universities? J High Educ Policy Manag 41(1):104–117
5. Radanović I, Likić R (2018) Opportunities for use of blockchain technology in medicine. Appl Health Econ Health Policy 16(5):583–590
6. Hoy MB (2017) An Introduction to the blockchain and its implications for libraries and medicine. Med Ref Serv Q 36(3):273–279
7. Transfer & Mobility–2018 (20182018) National student clearinghouse-research center. https://nscresearchcenter.org/signaturereport15/#:~:text=Out%20of%20all%20first%2Dtime, with%20a%20two%2Dyear%20credential
8. Sharples M, Domingue J (2016) The blockchain and kudos: a distributed system for educational record, reputation and reward. Springer International Publishing, Cham
9. Chen G et al (2018) Exploring blockchain technology and its potential applications for education. Smart Learn Environ 5(1):1
10. Swamy J, Parmar K (2020) Secure and decentralized academic transcript system based on blockchain technology, pp 345–351
11. Kosmarski A (2020) Blockchain adoption in academia: promises and challenges. J Open Innov Technol Market Complex 6(4):117
12. Turkanović M et al (2018) EduCTX: a blockchain-based higher education credit platform. IEEE Access 6:5112–5127
13. Mohan V (2019) On the use of blockchain-based mechanisms to tackle academic misconduct. Res Policy 48(9):103805

14. Fanelli D (2009) How many scientists fabricate and falsify research? A systematic review and meta-analysis of survey data. PLoS One 4(5):e5738
15. Rosamond B (2002) Plagiarism, academic norms and the governance of the profession. Politics 22(3):167–174
16. Khatoon A (2020) A blockchain-based smart contract system for healthcare management. Electronics 9(1):94
17. Dunn A (2020) More than 1,000 aspiring surgeons couldn't take a critical online exam after the system failed. Now they're left worried it may never happen. https://www.businessinsider.com/american-board-of-surgery-online-testing-plan-fails-2020-7#: ~ :text=An%20exam%20taken%20by%20surgeons,to%20a%20board%2Dcertified%20surgeon
18. ABS Issuing Refunds, Launching security investigation for virtual 2020 general surgery QE. https://www.absurgery.org/default.jsp?news_virtualgsqe07.17. Accessed February 28, 2021
19. Stawicki S et al (2019) Roadmap for the development of academic and medical applications of blockchain technology: joint statement from OPUS 12 global and litecoin cash foundation. J Emerg Trauma Shock 12(1):64–67

Distributed Research Networks

12

Thomas F. Heston and Alexandra Dullea

> *The blockchain symbolizes a shift in power from the centers to the edges of the networks.*
>
> —William Mougayar

Abstract

Successful medical research requires a fair and meticulous peer review process, safe and secure data storage, and verifiable statistical analysis. Initially, the medical research system utilized a centralized system to disseminate information. A centralized system is advantageous because of its ability for speedy dissemination of information; however, it is vulnerable to the influence of possible bias and offers a clear target for hackers. With technology advancements, the centralized system morphed into a decentralized model that encourages improved collaboration but can either foster innovation or limit the diversity of ideas depending on the circumstances. More recently, blockchain technology has made the advancement to a distributed network system possible. A distributed network is less vulnerable to hacking or corruption but slows down publication speed. This chapter will review the advantages and disadvantages of the three major types of networks (centralized, decentralized, and distributed), as well as propose a human-computer hybrid research network that could provide a solution for improving the quality and circulation of research. Such an approach would address the need for meticulous peer review by offering greater peer

T. F. Heston (✉) · A. Dullea
Department of Medical Education and Clinical Sciences, Washington State University, Spokane, WA, USA
e-mail: tom.heston@wsu.edu

T. F. Heston
Department of Family Medicine, University of Washington, Seattle, WA, USA

© The Author(s), under exclusive license to Springer Nature Switzerland AG 2023
S. Stawicki (ed.), *Blockchain in Healthcare*, Integrated Science 10,
https://doi.org/10.1007/978-3-031-14591-9_12

review rigor with a larger pool of peer reviewers available. Additionally, the implementation of such a network through a blockchain inscription method would allow for secure, long term data storage.

Keywords

Medical research · Blockchain technology · Peer review

Introduction

Bioethics demands that medical research be conducted in a rigorous manner that protects human subjects. Research findings must also undergo peer review to ensure that proper procedures are followed and that the interpretation of data requiring statistical analysis can be objectively verified by third parties. Following review, the research must be published and made readily available to medical professionals and the lay public. To meet these demands, data must be accurately collected, safely stored, and made available for re-evaluation by future scientists.

The communication of medical research initially followed a centralized network model where information flow was controlled by a central authority. Although there were multiple centralized networks, there was no collaboration between the central authorities. However, as communication technology advanced, there was greater opportunity for the central authorities to link up and form a minimally decentralized model, which is the current state of medical research. Now, with the development of blockchain technology, medical research can advance to a widely decentralized model, commonly known as a distributed network [1]. The advantages of a distributed network are numerous and include greater transparency, improved peer-review, and increased permanence of the data [2]. However, significant challenges remain. The protection of human subjects depends upon the thoughtful and thorough evaluation of research projects by an Institutional Review Board (IRB). In addition, peer review requires thoughtful analysis of manuscripts by experts in the specialty. These decisions are complex and are not currently amenable to a strict algorithmic approach.

In this chapter, the three major type of networks (centralized, decentralized, and distributed) will be discussed, and their advantages and disadvantages in terms of medical research will be reviewed. Finally, a human-computer hybrid network model will be proposed as a starting point for discussions to improve the quality and dissemination of medical research.

Centralized Networks

Centralized networks can be visualized using a hub and spoke model (Fig. 12.1). In this model, information from an outlying node must pass through a central node before reaching another node in the network. Nodes typically are thought of as individual computers, with the central node being the mainframe computer. This centralized node is also called a central authority. The central authority verifies data and regulates information flow. In clinical medicine, centralized networks are common. For example, teleradiology programs typically use a centralized network model, where images are obtained at outlying sites, then sent to a single authority that distributes the studies for interpretation by radiologists located at the hub site. In this system, information flow is strictly controlled, and all information is stored by the central authority.

When applied to medical research, some outlying nodes represent individual researchers who conduct their studies at numerous different institutions. Their research is sent directly via a spoke to a peer-reviewed medical journal, which is the network hub. The network hub receives information from researchers and then sends out approved research to the readers of the journal, which are also represented by outlying nodes. Thus, the network hubs control a bi-directional information flow, in that they receive/process research manuscripts from researchers and then send the selected peer-reviewed research out to readers via journal publication.

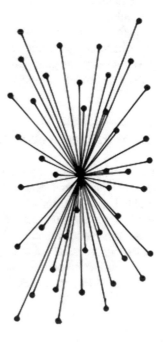

Fig. 12.1 In a centralized network, all nodes send and receive information from a single central authority that controls information flow. Outlying nodes are not able to directly communicate with each other (public domain image courtesy of freesvg.org)

Once a research manuscript is received by a journal, the editorial board, in most cases, is responsible for peer review (this may be delegated). The board reviews the manuscript and gives recommendations to the editor regarding the fitness of the studies and the overall appeal of the research. The editor then takes these recommendations and decides what research is worthy of publication. In a centralized network, the medical journal is the central authority with significant power over information flow. This power is typically highly concentrated, with just a few individuals making up the editorial board that gives recommendations on whether to publish a manuscript to the editor. However, the greatest concentration of power over information flow is held by a single individual, the journal editor, who makes the final decision regarding whether a study is suitable for publication.

The primary advantage of a centralized network is the speed of information flow. In all cases, the communication between any two outlying nodes is a simple two-step process: the first node sends information to the hub, which then sends the information to the second node. With a highly reliable, trusted central authority, the result is the rapid publication of high-quality research. However, centralized networks also have significant shortcomings. In medical research, their biggest disadvantage is the influence of bias on the central authority, since a single person is largely responsible for deciding what information will be disseminated and what information will be censored. For computer centralized networks, the greatest disadvantage is the vulnerability of a single computer from multiple threats such as hardware failures, unauthorized data access, or data corruption from hackers. As it pertains to research publication, the central hub has several human vulnerabilities. Editors may steer scientific opinion by only publishing research they are interested in, regardless of scientific rigor. Editors can be caught up in broad political issues and publish research they believe will have an impact on current politics. They may publish sensational research, in spite of low scientific rigor, because of the notoriety from increased coverage by the lay press. In sort, journal editors have incredible power over what gets published, and their individual weaknesses can adversely impact the broader scientific community [3].

Decentralized Networks

Decentralized networks are more complex than centralized networks in that there are multiple linked central authorities that control information flow. In a decentralized network, individual, outlying nodes still communicate with the larger network via a central authority; however, multiple central authorities from various centralized networks are linked together. Therefore, information flow is still controlled via a central authority, but collaboration between multiple central authorities is allowed. A common example of a decentralized network is the system of airport hubs for airline travel (Fig. 12.2).

Fig. 12.2 In a decentralized
network, a small number of
central authorities collaborate
with each other to control
information flow. Information
from outlying nodes must go
through a central authority
prior to transmission to a
different outlying node
(public domain image
courtesy of freesvg.org)

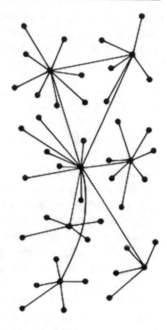

The publication of medical research has loosely evolved to follow a decentralized network model. For example, journal editors, as individual central authorities, not only control what research gets published in their own journal but can also influence what gets published in other similar journals. This is done via an informal type of collaboration where editors get together to make uniform decisions that affect multiple medical journals. This collaboration is commonly accomplished through the establishment of industry standards, such as recommendations for conflict of interest disclosures [4].

The primary advantage of decentralized networks is the speed of information transmission combined with the ability to improve information quality due to the collaboration of central authorities. However, this can become a significant weakness if the collaboration turns into collusion. Central authorities, with time, can become susceptible to groupthink, and, in the case of medical research, the biases of individual journal editors can be amplified by this collaboration/collusion. Therefore, unorthodox revolutionary research may be erroneously rejected or suppressed, resulting in the slower advancement of medical science.

Although they are an improvement over centralized hub-and-spoke networks, decentralized networks nevertheless impede the flow of information by mandating a central authority. For example, although there are multiple social media central authorities on the Internet, such as Twitter, YouTube, and Facebook, these central authorities often work together and collude to block certain ideas or personalities. Thus, information and ideas can be censored by a small number of authorities (usually highly controlled by a single person) and, on the flip side, propaganda or favored ideas can be promoted by these same central authorities. Unfortunately, the current state of medical research has a similar structural foundation and is subject to both the strengths and weaknesses of having central authorities decide what research to publish and what research to reject.

Distributed Networks

Highly decentralized networks are known as distributed networks. These networks have no central authority and no centralized network of hubs. The hallmark of distributed networks is the lack of a central authority alongside a method of maintaining data integrity. This is the fundamental feature of blockchain technology. In this model, there is no ability for an individual or small group of central authorities to control data verification or information flow. Nodes have multiple connections with other nodes, and any single node may join or leave the network at will without affecting the overall function of the network. Moreover, whereas centralized and lightly decentralized networks can be visualized in two dimensions, the interconnections in a distributed network are much more complex (Fig. 12.3).

While information flow in a distributed network may be less efficient compared to a centralized or lightly decentralized network, resistance to data corruption can be greatly increased. Whereas the corruption of a single central authority (or small

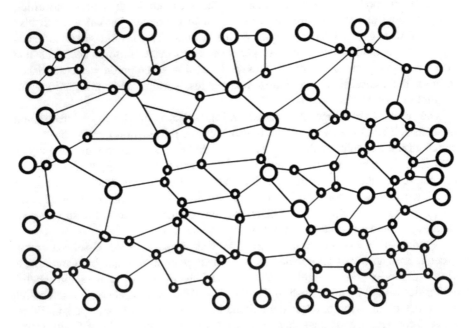

Fig. 12.3 In a distributed network, there is no central authority, and thus no opportunity for a restricted collaboration by a small number of nodes to control information flow (public domain image courtesy of freesvg.org)

group of central authorities) will break down a centralized (or decentralized) network, distributed networks, as implemented by blockchain technology, require a large proportion of all nodes to be corrupt before the network fails. The problem of overcoming corrupt nodes has been described as the Byzantine Generals Problem [5], and the solution set forth by Satoshi Nakamoto (the Bitcoin network), combines cryptography with proof of work in a manner highly resistant to node corruption [6]. In short, instead of trusting a central authority to ensure data integrity, the network as a whole becomes the means of ensuring data integrity. The transparency alone makes it more resistant to human biases [7].

Although personal information is highly encrypted, the Bitcoin network and most cryptocurrency networks are open and transparent. This has the effect of making them less, not more, susceptible to nodal corruption. For example, egregious acts of bias that would be readily detected in a public forum can go undetected when committed in private. Thus, a single corrupt journal editor can cause a widespread propagation of biased research, and go completely undetected.

Distributed networks negate the effect of a single corrupt editor. Distributed networks are open and transparent. Any biases are committed in public, and thus are quickly detected. The ability of a rogue editor to impede high quality research publication, or to infect scientific research with personal biases is non-existent. It is harder to commit editorial misconduct when using a transparent distributed network process, and easier to commit editorial misconduct behind the closed doors of a boardroom.

Despite individual cryptocurrency wallets and exchanges having been compromised, the Bitcoin network itself has not been hacked, primarily due to the complexity of cryptography. This is a profound testament to the resilience of the Bitcoin network, given a market capitalization of over $1 trillion USD. This is a tremendous bounty for hackers, yet the Bitcoin network itself remains uncorrupted in spite of theoretical vulnerabilities [8]. Perhaps the biggest threat is from the development of quantum computers, yet even this is thought to be unlikely to break cryptocurrencies [9, 10]. Using soft forks in the software, distributed networks can upgrade their cryptography to keep pace with new developments. Furthermore, cryptographic schemes resistant to quantum computing are being actively developed [11].

A primary advantage of transparent distributed networks, secured by cryptography, is greater data integrity and resistance to corruption. This improvement comes primarily at the cost of slower data transmission speeds. For computer systems, dramatic advances in fiber optic and wireless data speeds makes this slower transmission of data negligible.

Medical research could benefit from the features of a distributed network. The transparency would increase trust in the process by both scientists and the lay public. Cryptography would ensure data integrity and proper credit be given to researchers. A pure computer based distributed network, however, would not be sufficient in solving the complexities of research publication because of the inflexibility of a purely mathematical algorithmic approach.

Human–Computer Hybrid Research Networks

Medical research requires the uncompromising protection of human subjects by an IRB. Research must also be rigorously evaluated to ensure that proper scientific principles were followed during the data collection and analysis. The complexity of these tasks requires human oversight of medical research to ensure ethical compliance with universally agreed upon standards [12]. Human judgment is necessary to protect human interests [13].

At the outset of a research project, the proposal is first presented to an IRB. This process would not change in a hybrid research distributed network, although individual IRBs could theoretically form a distributed network with the sole purpose of approving or rejecting research protocols. Indeed, a blockchain type of distributed research network would not replace institutional oversight of research being actively performed. However, when research has been completed and is ready for publication, the manuscript would be presented to a human-computer hybrid distributed network. Consensus regarding a manuscript's suitability for publication could then be achieved using any of a variety of protocols, such as proof of work or proof of stake. When consensus is achieved, the raw data and manuscript would then be published to a public blockchain.

One advantage of utilizing a distributed network for the peer review and publication of medical research is greater rigor regarding peer review. With an open, transparent network that requires consensus, the pool of peer reviewers would be much larger than an individual journal could reach. This larger pool of peer reviewers would help prevent mistakes from being made during a rush to publication during emergencies. Enthusiasm and pressurized research can create mistakes through the introduction of shortcuts in research standards and researchers working outside of their field of expertise [14]. In addition, rushing to publication in times of health crises can adversely impact the scientific peer review of research, resulting in the publication of low-quality research and the retraction of research articles only after they have adversely affected the public. For example, approximately 6 months into the Covid-19 pandemic, 37 research publications about Covid-19 had already been retracted [15]. Clearly, the existing methods of peer review have much to be desired.

Blockchains can consist of closed, proprietary networks or open, fully transparent networks. Cryptocurrency implementations of blockchain technology are almost universally open and transparent networks. For Bitcoin, its mechanism for ensuring data integrity and avoiding the double-spend problem is proof of work. Nodes that ensure data integrity (miners) engage in mathematical work on a problem that is difficult to solve but easy to verify. The first node to solve the problem gets a reward, then after the solution has been verified, a consensus is reached. The entire network then moves on to solving the next problem [16]. A human-computer hybrid distributed network would similarly require a consensus protocol, with the data being routed by the computer network but the work of ensuring data integrity being performed by humans.

In addition to their ability to maintain data integrity, blockchain open encryption methods have a proven track record of data security and can help protect private information. This is critical, because in spite of well-intentioned privacy policies, health data is valuable data that strongly attracts hackers. In the last quarter of 2018, for example, an analysis of Fortune 500 companies found that pharmaceutical companies were the most targeted group with an average of 71 attacks per business [17]. DNA analysis companies are particularly rich targets for hackers, yet they often do not live up to the policies set forth in their privacy statements [18]. Private storage of medical information can also be highly influenced by market economics. For example, Fitbit wearable devices openly state that they transmit information to corporate affiliates that provide them global services including sales, marketing, *and research* [19]. Although it is emphasized that "personally identifiable" data is kept private, users must trust a single corporation (a central authority) with their personal information, ultimately depending upon the reliability of a single person, the Chief Privacy Officer.

Along with security concerns, traditional methods of data storage can experience issues with long-term accessibility. For example, storing data long-term on microfiche or paper is problematic because it can be easily destroyed by a single fire. Furthermore, private data repositories, such as Amazon Web Services, can arbitrarily decide to delete data that they (as central authorities) deem inappropriate. Furthermore, these private storage sites are susceptible to collusion in banning data [20]. Private storage methods also have low availability to a global audience, which limits the independent analysis of the data.

In contrast to private data storage, blockchains store data in a transparent and immutable manner, and they are perhaps the best way to store data for long periods of time. Furthermore, a research blockchain network would not be able to ban data once a peer review consensus is reached. Nodes in such a distributed network would be incentivized to maintain the data through the provision of storage and retrieval fees. There are also several existing blockchain projects that provide an alternative to centralized cloud-based services. These peer-to-peer networks capitalize on the fact that approximately half of the world's file storage space is unused. Current implementations of distributed peer-to-peer file storage networks include Filecoin, Storj, and Siacoin. All utilize a cryptocurrency token to incentivize data storage, as agreed upon in a smart contract. Although these projects all are in their infancy, their shared objective is to provide file storage at a lower cost, with higher security, and greater long-term reliability. This is an ideal situation for research data, making it available for analysis by future researchers as technology and medical knowledge advances.

Conclusion

Currently, the publication and dissemination of medical research is controlled primarily by a relatively small group of journal editors, the central authorities of hub and spoke networks. Therefore, the regulation of research information flow heavily depends upon the reliability, integrity, and trustworthiness of just a few people. While the integrity of journal editors may be beyond reproach, this centralized control has the effect of amplifying personal biases and exposing specific focal points for hackers. In contrast, the evolution of a research publishing model based upon a distributed rather than a centralized network has the advantages of more robust peer review, greater immutability of raw research data, improved transparency, wider information dissemination, and stronger data privacy. Furthermore, a human-computer hybrid distributed research network would create consensus through the work of human peer reviewers. Data storage, privacy, and information flow would be accomplished through peer-to-peer storage, modern cryptography, and a transparent distributed computer network. Indeed, blockchain technology provides all the necessary tools to implement an improved global system that will ensure the wide availability of high-quality medical research.

References

1. Deer M (2022) Centralized vs decentralized digital networks: Key differences. Cointelegraph [cited 2022 Sep 15].Available from: https://cointelegraph.com/explained/centralized-vs-decentralized-digital-networks-key-differences
2. Heston TF (2017) The blockchain-based scientific study. Digit Med 3(2):66–68
3. Barbour V, Astaneh B, Irfan M (2016) Challenges in publication ethics. Ann R Coll Surg Engl 98(4):241–243
4. Pickar JH (2019) Conflicts of interest and the ICMJE disclosure form. Climacteric 22(3):215–216
5. Lamport L, Shostak R, Pease M (1982) The Byzantine generals problem. ACM Trans Program Lang Syst 4(3):382–401
6. Nakamoto S (2008) Bitcoin: a peer-to-peer electronic cash system [Internet]. Bitcoin.org. [cited 2018 Jun 7]. Available from: https://bitcoin.org/bitcoin.pdf
7. Kakarlapudi PV, Mahmoud QH (2021) A systematic review of blockchain for consent management. Healthcare (Basel) 9(2)
8. Baldwin W (2020) Can all of bitcoin be hacked? [Internet]. Forbes. [cited 2021 Feb 14]. Available from: https://www.forbes.com/sites/baldwin/2020/02/16/can-all-of-bitcoin-be-hacked/?sh=637c3f3f1dc1
9. Huang R (2020) Here's why quantum computing will not break cryptocurrencies [Internet]. Forbes. [cited 2021 Feb 15]. Available from: https://www.forbes.com/sites/rogerhuang/2020/12/21/heres-why-quantum-computing-will-not-break-cryptocurrencies/?sh=5f0416c9167b
10. Chirgwin R (2016) SHA3–256 is quantum-proof, should last billions of years [Internet]. The Register. [cited 2021 Feb 15]. Available from: https://www.theregister.com/2016/10/18/sha3256_good_for_beelions_of_years_say_boffins/
11. Mavroeidis V, Vishi K, DM, Jøsang A (2018) The impact of quantum computing on present cryptography. Ijacsa 9(3)
12. DuBois JM (2004) Is compliance a professional virtue of researchers? Reflections on promoting the responsible conduct of research. Ethics Behav 14(4):383–395

13. Gillette C (2020) Do mandatory minimums increase racial disparities in federal criminal sentencing? Undergr Econ Rev 17(1)
14. Doroshow D, Podolsky S, Barr J (2020) Biomedical research in times of emergency: lessons from history. Ann Intern Med 173(4):297–299
15. Solbakk JH, Bentzen HB, Holm S, Heggestad AKT, Hofmann B, Robertsen A et al (2020) Back to WHAT? The role of research ethics in pandemic times. Med Health Care Philos
16. Bach LM, Mihaljevic B, Zagar M (2018) Comparative analysis of blockchain consensus algorithms. 2018 41st international convention on information and communication technology, electronics and microelectronics (MIPRO). IEEE, pp 1545–1550
17. Davis J (2018) Pharmaceutical companies most targeted industry by cybercriminals [Internet]. Health IT Security. [cited 2021 Feb 14]. Available from: https://healthitsecurity.com/news/pharmaceutical-companies-most-targeted-industry-by-cybercriminals
18. Aldhous P, Reilly M (2009) How my genome was hacked. New Scientist 201(2701):6–9
19. Fitbit Legal Privacy Policy [Internet]. [cited 2021 Feb 15]. Available from: https://www.fitbit.com/global/us/legal/privacy-policy
20. Fitzpatrick A (2021) AWS parler ban is a big deal for the future of the internet [Internet]. Time. [cited 2021 Feb 14]. Available from: https://time.com/5929888/amazon-parler-aws/

Use of Blockchain Technology for Implantable Medical Device Tracking

Kristofer S. Matullo, Chad A. Amato, and Pavel Burskii

> *The future belongs to those who seize the opportunities created by innovation.*
>
> —Delos M. Cosgrove, MD

Abstract

A blockchain is an auspicious tool in the era of technological advancements. As a form of horizontal innovation, blockchain technology will drastically change the healthcare industry in consecutive years, addressing health information exchange's main problematic points, such as varying data standards, inconsistent rules and permissions, security breaches, and high data transmission costs [1]. While blockchain certainly is not a one cure for all solution, it does offer a new distributed framework to magnify and boost the integration of health care information amongst a range of uses and participants. This chapter aims to

K. S. Matullo (✉) · C. A. Amato
Department of Orthopedic Surgery, St. Luke's University Health Network, Bethlehem, PA, USA
e-mail: kristofer.matullo@sluhn.org

C. A. Amato
e-mail: chad.amato@sluhn.org

K. S. Matullo
Lewis Katz School of Medicine at, Temple University, Bethlehem, PA, USA

P. Burskii
Department of Research and Innovation, St. Luke's University Health Network, Bethlehem, PA, USA
e-mail: pavelburskii@gmail.com

review current blockchain technology applications, particularly in implantable medical devices, raising awareness about this technology and promoting future interest in that topic for the research community.

Keywords

Decentralization · Interoperability · Traceability · Transparency · Supply chain · Distributed ledger · Data security · Smart contracts

Introduction

According to Peter Diamandis, MD (X Prize Foundation), technology is changing the world mainly through three primary mechanisms: democratization (easier access), demonetization (decreasing the cost), and dematerialization (converting information into a digital format). All innovative technology goes through a period of deception before ultimately becoming disruptive" [1].

With the most recent news that for the first time, orders for medical devices were successfully processed via blockchain in Swiss hospitals [2], humanity is making a new step towards data unification and interoperability. Several initiatives worldwide have already been accomplished ensuring the safety and integrity of electronic health records, digital prescriptions, and images, resulting in cost reduction, more effective management of the supply chain, and proper tracking of resources with authentication options [3].

As we already know, a blockchain is a continuously growing list of records, called blocks, which are linked and secured using two-way encryption. Each block typically contains a cryptographic hash of the previous block, a timestamp, and transaction data [4]. By design, blockchain is inherently resistant to modification of the data. It is an open distributed ledger that can record transactions between two parties efficiently and in a verifiable and permanent way. In other words, both parties can prove whether data is valid, given that the data is stored appropriately [5]. That decreases the need for a trusted mediator and increases the end-user independence from the third party ("middleman"), allowing more efficient control of privacy—a matter of primary importance in healthcare.

The properties mentioned above are essential in the medical device industry, where blockchain technology can unleash its full potential, successfully meeting the four efficiency criteria proposed in the paper published by Deloitte [6].

1. There is a need for a database where multiple participants can generate transactions that change the shared repository information.
2. Parties need to trust if transactions are valid.
3. Intermediaries are inefficient or not trusted as an arbiter of truth.
4. Enhanced security is needed to ensure the integrity of the system.

While used in that way, blockchain technology will improve healthcare's digital environment, making it more compatible for workers and convenient for patients. It promises to increase monetization values and expand the trust-based business environment, thus transition the industry towards an ultimate patient-oriented ecosystem.

What Exactly Blockchain Technology Means for Implantable Medical Devices?

When investigating this question, we will review blockchain technology applications separated into the three main domain:

1. Health Information Exchange and Device Tracking.
2. Smart Contracts.
3. Medical Device Development.

Then we will discuss each domain from the standpoint of, arguably, the most faster-moving healthcare segments adopting the blockchain technology:

1. Data Management.
2. Clinical Trials.
3. Supply Chain Management.

Methods

Relevant studies published after January 2015 were selected for review with an extensive electronic search using Google Scholar, PubMed/Medline, Trip, and Microsoft Academic engines. Academic literature, grey literature, industry publications, and related media sources were reviewed while preparing this article by authors. The search was performed using the following terms: *blockchain, medical device, tracking, implants, smart contracts, supply chain*, and their combinations. Studies that evaluated and proposed applications of blockchain technology in tracking medical devices were considered. Studies were excluded if they were not accessible in the English language if the full text was unavailable. Additionally, the most prominent stakeholders engaged in exploring blockchain solutions for the medical device industry were identified and described. This chapter aims to fill the gap between IT-focused manuscripts about the technology itself and the literature that primarily reviews applications in the pharma industry or is devoted solely to potential economic impact. Here, we attempt to summarize the available data for tracking medical devices and find out gaps in knowledge needed to be addressed before further conclusions regarding the use of blockchain technology can be drawn.

Health Information Exchange and Device Tracking

Data acquired from implantable, wearable, or monitoring devices falling under the same category from the blockchain aspect. It is a technological challenge for healthcare organizations, professionals, policymakers, and payors and an existing concern for patients' privacy and safety. As confirmed in recently published articles describing the vulnerability of cardioverter-defibrillators [7, 8] and infusion pumps for cyberattacks [9], a potential intruder can modify a device's program regimen, potentially leading to patient harm from rapid battery depletion, inappropriate pace administration [10], or manipulations with drug infusion rates. Responding to these challenges, the FDA recently developed a pilot blockchain-based platform to exchange health data between EHR, trials, and wearable medical devices, attempting to test this solution security against existing alternatives [11]. Medical devices' safety and quality are directly related to a patient's life, and such high risks determine the necessity to create an effectively operable system with traceability. Tracking medical devices prevents the basis for making counterfeit or unqualified products market-ready and helps companies find the source of the problem, control quality, and safety, and effectively work with devices' generated data. Figure 13.1 graphically represents blockchain technology opportunities for medical device data management.

The blockchain's decentralized nature presumes that no single authority controls the information, allowing all participants, from the regulators to the end-users, to secure and access information in its accuracy. Because a limited amount of information can be stored on one block of a chain (1 Mb) [6], it has to *supplement* existing electronic health records (EHR) to increase data exchange interoperability. Current EHR systems hold large volumes of abstract data such as MRI images, various monitoring data, etc. [12]. This type of stored information would require specific pointers leading to "on-chain" data from a separate "off-chain" server and

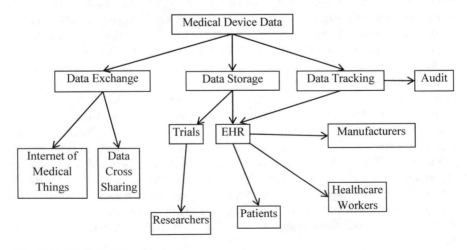

Fig. 13.1 Medical device data tree

in that way, achieving disintermediation of trust and eliminating the need for brokered data operators because all participants would have access to the distributed ledger to maintain and secure information exchange [13]. Let us bring the example of blockchain application in the storage and exchange of data generated by the interaction of patient's medical devices and the Internet of Medical Things technology (IoMT). In the patient with a history of type 1 diabetes mellitus and implanted continuous glucose monitor, who recently was diagnosed with an arrhythmia and discharged with the monitoring device, all data, including heart rhythm, blood glucose, blood oxygen levels, and amount of insulin administered via smartpen can be safely transmitted and stored via one platform allowing access to information for multiple care teams [14]. The patient or provider can issue a private key that could automatically and securely record a patient's blood glucose levels and then communicate with an automated insulin delivery device to maintain blood glucose at healthy intervals. This technology would allow for information to be tracked by patients and providers in real-time with an option which part of data can be hidden and which part can be distributed [15]. Blockchain infrastructure for the IoMT could manage health data from wearable and temporarily or permanently implantable devices with enhanced safety and productivity [16].

Cross-institutional sharing will significantly increase clinical trials' efficiency and continuity of care through data access from multiple health care institutions [17]. Shared data enables synchronization and fast updates across the network, maintaining transparency where data located and who have access to it. The blockchain has the flexibility to make data visible or hidden (e.g., password protected) depending on the user's target goals and authorization rights. In that way, blockchain technology will ensure sensitive data is protected from breaches [18].

"The current state of health care records is disjointed and stovepiped due to lack of common architectures and standards [6]". Consequently, increasing amounts of the paper trail (digitalized or analog), from manufacturer to implanting physician, creates a burden affecting care delivery and continuity, increasing data transaction costs, and compromising easy data access. A provided example can become more complicated if the implanting physician and follow-up provider are different, or when the patient relocates, or when there is a need to trace multiple devices or components in use. All these factors can be slowing down the efficiency of health information exchange. Blockchain technology, on the contrary, can ensure data integrity and establish a record of the device usage via linked hashes and public/private key pair cryptography, which can be used for storing different parts and subsections of the EHR (or pointers to it) on the blockchain, and be available across multiple healthcare systems [19].

A public blockchain can act as an access control manager to the healthcare records stored on a private blockchain or to the "off-chain" data [20]. This model will allow data access through a user's unique identifier following an encrypted link to each transaction's health record with a timestamp. It is crucial to notice that blockchain serves as an immutable audit log where data queried on the chain is tracked to ensure that only authorized users can access it. Therefore any interaction within the chained data instantly becomes known to all participants and requires

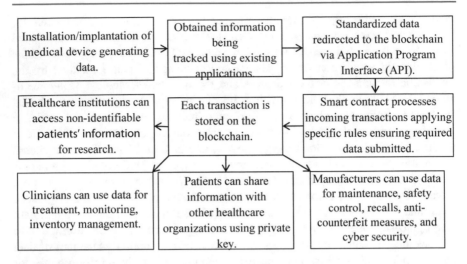

Fig. 13.2 Flowchart for medical device data processing

authorization by the network before new information can be added, creating "trustless" collaboration while simultaneously recording an immutable audit of all interactions [21]. Figure 13.2 is a flowchart that represents the blockchain technology application for medical device data management using the framework model described in Deloitte's report [6].

The existing medical device tracking system is based on a server-client model and integrates Internet of Things technology with a radio frequency identification system (RFID) [22]. However, when thousands of IoT devices are connected, limitations and issues with synchronization may arise. This area represents another opportunity where blockchain technology can be utilized. Several recent studies confirmed that RFID-enabled healthcare management proves its usefulness and provides clear monetary savings with optimizing the hospital workflow [23, 24]. Adding the blockchain approach to RFID tracking creates additional benefits over traditional solutions, the most prominent of which is decentralization and immutability. The blockchain consensus mechanism coupled with storage and encrypted distribution can help prevent unauthorized access by tampering with data and function [25]. The basic architecture of such a platform proposed in the study by Xiaoling Xia et al. can be divided into six layers: data, network, consensus, incentive, contract, and application layers [26].

Blockchain technology is mainly used in the data layer, network layer, consensus layer, and application layer. The data layer is responsible for distributed storage of the collected data on blockchain nodes. The network layer will disseminate verified data amongst the network. All device parameters, including location, patients data, status, service, and authentification for the entire lifecycle of the device, will be connected to the specific encrypted node ID number. Huh, et al. suggests that intercommunication in such a system should occur through an Ethereum blockchain using RSA encrypted public key system. The device's public key is stored on the blockchain, and the associated private key is stored within the device [27]. The consensus layer uses the Practical Byzantine Tolerant Protocol (PBFT), ensuring the safe distribution of data amongst the blockchain nodes. The application layer is responsible for user interfaces where manufacturers, regulators, and hospitals can interact with the device and its data. Initially, the device manufacturer registering an account in the system, authenticity is verified by the administrator, and the system automatically assigns the corresponding pair of keys. The manufacturer identifies all devices and generates individual electronic files for each. The final product can be distributed to the end-users via a traceable supply chain where all participants, including hospitals and patients, can obtain relevant device information in its safety and integrity using RFID [26].

Smart Contracts

Healthcare is one of the world's leading industries by the number of traditional formal contracts involved in its functioning. The contracts are made between patients and hospitals, hospitals and healthcare organizations, manufacturers, insurance companies, etc. Smart contracts are special algorithms of code stored on the blockchain that automatically execute functions when customizable and predetermined conditions are met, allowing the start of events, exchanging values, and transfer of information. Smart contracts are the unique and most promising properties of blockchain technology meant to streamline the process of making traditional contracts between parties "encased" in the blockchain, thus eliminating several participating intermediaries [28]. It is worth noting that this feature does not altogether abolish the necessity of trust. Instead, it puts the traditional form of interaction on the next level, creating an opportunity for multiple parties' target goals to exist on one unified and automatically enforced function [29]. Figure 13.3 graphically represents smart contract opportunities for medical devices.

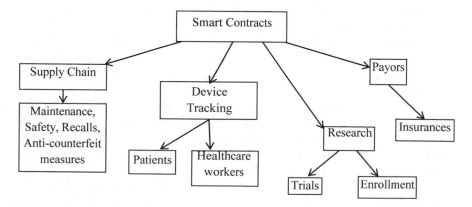

Fig. 13.3 Smart contracts application tree

A smart contract acting as a superstructure for a blockchain-based system can further strengthen and improve its efficiency. The receiving party can verify the proposed record before accepting or rejecting the data, thus keeping participants informed and creates an evident and transparent chain of custody.

Let us describe a process of use of blockchain technology to track and trace medical devices from the manufacturer to the patient and further. Data management based on smart contracts creates opportunities to track the entire end-to-end process from raw materials and manufacturing to implantation or installation processes to the device's final utilization or recycling [30]. Moreover, information and control on manufacturing locations, inventory capacity, shipping and expiration dates, storage temperature and humidity—everything could be kept and monitored on the blockchain. The decentralized and immutable nature of technology will help minimize fraud and counterfeit of medical devices. Assuming that there are no third parties involved in the device supply chain, it will reduce participants' vulnerability to scam. In addition to tracking finished products, the entire directory of approved parts and components of the medical device—Bill of Materials (BOM) can be maintained on the tamperproof record. Many manufacturing, quality, and service information on Device History Record (DHR) can be securely stored on blockchain where it cannot be altered but can be quickly accessed in the case of recall or safety concerns. If the device has failed, the on-chain record could help precisely determine if there were manufacturing issues, interference on its way to the patient, misuse of the device, and what circumstances can lead to an error, allowing to generate root-cause analyses more effectively. The blockchain could track devices also after their use to ensure they were disposed or reprocessed appropriately.

One of the researchers' most significant challenges today is finding the right patient for the trial matching project's requirements. Approximately 80% of trials fail to meet the initial enrollment target [31]. That type of work involves much manual time-consuming labor when mapping parameters of interest in the EHR. Even though the current state of EHR's data indexation for search is far more advanced than it was several years ago, it still presents a significant challenge for effective operations. Additionally, every manual work is prone to errors and human factor issues, especially when multiple EHR systems are involved. Because smart contracts are automated functions, the trial's potential participants will be suggested by the system as soon as they are registered and parameters of interest are detected. Since blockchain records cannot be registered without validation, researchers can gather large and specific samples of participants, ensuring that the required subjects are getting in.

From the patient's perspective, smart contracts make it easier to know the pertinent details about implanted device functions, current status, measurable parameters, required maintenance dates, and what data is transmitted to the healthcare provider. Blockchain can also help with compliance and proper device use via the "proof of action" function, where patients are automatically notified and can electronically verify their adherence to the prescribed regimens, diet, etc. Moreover, it is possible to create built-in algorithms with optional incentives for patients corresponding to their interactions with the device [32]. The smart contract will also allow patients to eliminate the vast majority of paperwork and upload single medical forms or requests on the blockchain network, sending them directly to physicians they visit.

Blockchain removes third-party payment services allowing payers and providers to negotiate claims tied to the value of care. Healthcare payments sent and received are immediately getting distributed between all the smart contract participants. It becomes easier for insurance companies to access patients' ledger with the record of all services provided, ensuring paid claims' efficiency and accuracy [33]. The potential for applications is vast. Automatic payments and the transfer of values once conditions are met will transform the industry. For example payor's smart contract can send the payment as soon as shipment, installation, implantation, or maintenance of devices is recorded on the blockchain. Therefore, the roles of traditional intermediaries will be significantly changed.

Medical Device Development

This section will review essential changes that blockchain technology can bring into the development of medical devices. Figure 13.4 graphically represents areas in which it can have the most impact.

Assuming that the data processed via blockchain becomes more protected and can be reviewed throughout the device lifecycle, the policymakers eventually will adjust regulations simplifying the process of approving new technologies creating a more significant influx of data for developers to work on and more time to spend on development rather than on documentation and audit [34]. Manufacturing and maintenance will also be streamlined with blockchain traceability function creating opportunities for easy collaboration on product requirements, architecture, and design via shared device master (DMR) and history records (DHR) [19].

Documentation supporting current medical device development is a hybrid of paper and electronic-based documentation. As this system moves from paper to shared electronic record format applying blockchain technology with traceability and electronic signature functions will help securely manage these documents. Finished products and devices participating in trials can exchange depersonalized

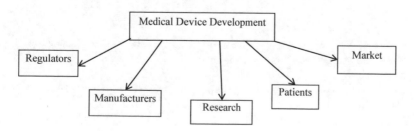

Fig. 13.4 Medical device development tree

patient data with researchers to compare the efficiency of various treatment protocols and device functions. Policymakers and regulators can use this data to work on guidelines or during the device certification process. Because all recorded data is transparent, it will significantly decrease the chances to certify a device that does not prove effective. Blockchain technology also has enormous potential to improve postmarket surveillance of medical devices. As regulators continuously raising safety standards, the amount of data for analysis growing exponentially. Blockchain technology, in that case, may support a more proactive approach to gather postmarket surveillance data where adverse event details can be generated automatically without the risk of omitting and compromising valuable data, decreasing the need for human interaction and eventually leading to a better quality of collected information [35].

Any regulatory or approval process based on neutrality and transparency is the most effective one. A blockchain solution for device development and certification will significantly increase the industry's fair and transparent competency while keeping patient safety a top priority. Patients, in their turn, will decide who can use their data and can choose to participate in the development of new personalized treatment options and even monetizing their health data by sharing it [36, 37]. Most patients are still unaware that their medical information is shared. Some companies already propose solutions for the patients, allowing them to control who owns their data and, potentially, find someone who wants to buy it with an agreement. These are beneficial aspects of technology that can help both parties, with financial incentives for patients and valuable data for device manufacturers. Examples of medical devices where blockchain technology can be successfully applied are illustrated in Table 13.1.

The implementation difficulty mentioned in the table above was assessed using the framework suggested by Lansiti et al. [33] and the global patterns of technology adoption. Device tracking and supply chain management are considered

Table 13.1 Blockchain applicability and implementation difficulty

Implantable medical devices	Examples	Blockchain Applicability	Implementation difficulty [33]
Sensory and Neurological	Intraocular lenses, cochlear implants, neurostimulators	Yes	High
Cardiovascular	Stents, valves, cardioverter-defibrillators, pacemakers	Yes	High
Orthopedic	Joints, pins, rods, screws, plates, etc	Yes	Moderate
Cosmetic	Prosthesis, Cosmetic implants	Yes	Low
Contraception	IUD	Yes	Low
Other organs and systems	Artificial sphincters, surgical mesh, continuous glucose monitors, infusion pumps, etc	Yes	High

low-novelty, low-coordination because they will be based on existed solutions as a base structure and most likely will proceed to the implementation processes relatively quickly. The difficulty of adapting the next steps will be based on the relation of technology novelty and efforts required for implementation and coordination. For example, adding smart contracts to the blockchain-based EHR system targeting specific medical device parameters requires substituting existing EHR with blockchain-based solutions and adding smart contracts as an additional function. It can be made achievable only in the case where blockchain will completely replace existing solutions. The degree of a novelty will be moderate since the basic EHR architecture already exists, but coordination efforts for such projects are significant and time-consuming. The industry's complete transformation when blockchain technology for medical devices will reach its maximum potential will take decades from now. It is not easy to predict, considering the adoption requires coordination of many participants from political, industrial, social, and legal spheres. To summarize, single-use applications like implantable device tracking are achievable in the near future, but the transformative phase, unfortunately, exists as a long-term goal on the roadmap.

Discussion

Blockchain presents numerous opportunities for implantable medical devices today; however, this technology is just starting its way to industry transformation. One of the most promising properties, its interoperability, ironically, remains uncertain, similarly as it is with interoperability of healthcare data overall at the current moment. Additionally, several potential disadvantages exist compared with the traditional approach to device data tracking and storage. The security vulnerabilities at the bottleneck points of blockchain may play a significant role in increasing security threats, including potential issues with personally identifiable data breaches, corruption of data stored in the digital ledger, improper use of smart contracts, etc. [38]. While data stored within the blockchain can be deidentified, the distributed access to the entire data set does have the risk of potential compromise and reidentification if a potential intruder gains access to more than 33.3–51% of chain nodes. Another point of concern is data processing times. The maximum rate of the transaction within the bitcoin networks is seven transactions per second [39], which can be a problem for large healthcare data networks. Platforms like Etherium are working to address this issue, but, as of now, blockchain technology is not optimized for high-volume data that need absolute privacy and instantaneous access within a single organization. Healthcare is a complex ecosystem where medical device operation consists of interactions between various stakeholders, including patients, providers, regulators, and payors. Each has specific goals and points of view, which makes agreements on unifying standards challenging. Health authorities should develop international standardized documents and policies on how data supposed to be sorted, stored, and exchanged in blockchain applications.

Blockchain technology cannot unleash its full potential if data exchange systems are not fully integrated. Another significant challenge is behavioral or human factors [40]. Assuming that the medical device industry is moving towards digitization very gradually, it will take a significant amount of time to convince some stakeholders to switch. Due to the current system's general conservatism and relatively slow adoption rate of new technologies in medicine, a significant shift has to happen before blockchain can be introduced broadly. The monetary cost of creating, using, and maintaining the blockchain infrastructure is another point for discussion. The cost of computing power is equal to volume multiplied by the size of transactions exchanged throughout the network per unit of time. Therefore it is hard to forecast the possible costs of applied blockchain technology accurately. Due to the limited workforce and resources in that field now, it is relatively expensive to implement technology [41] widely. Solid knowledge with a complete understanding of possible challenges coupled with continuous work on that topic will ultimately lead to the use of blockchain technology in medical devices.

Conclusion

Blockchain technology opens new horizons in healthcare and is intended to reduce complexity, enable trustless collaboration, and create secure and immutable information exchange [6]. Currently, it is proving usefulness in the non-healthcare industries. Lansiti et al. provide an example with TCP/IP protocol as an analogy to understand the current standpoint of blockchain [33]. The implementation patterns and chronology of both technologies can be similar. Just as e-mail enables bilateral communication, blockchain enables the bilateral exchange of values and contracts. Started on an enthusiastic basis in October 2008, similarly to TCP/IP, blockchain's core software is growing but still maintained by the volunteers' teams. Like an e-mail technology some time ago dramatically increased the speed and volume of exchanged information, the same pattern can be predicted for blockchain. The first widely used application of this technology in healthcare is most likely expected in the medical devices supply chain, where it will gradually decrease the need for human intervention bringing accountability, traceability, and transparency [42] in the field. The opportunities of blockchain technology are almost infinite. However, its applications' reliability, security, and cost-effectiveness require further research before practical implementation. Ideally, blockchain can revolutionize the medical devices industry and become an essential part of it, creating an internationally accessible system with reduced fraud, errors, delays, and optimized inventory management sealed with consumers' and partners' trust—the most crucial question "When?" for now, unfortunately, is not clear.

References

1. Bates Ramirez V (2016) The 6 Ds of tech disruption: a guide to the digital economy. https://singularityhub.com/2016/11/22/the-6-ds-of-tech-disruption-a-guide-to-the-digital-economy. Accessed 1 March 2021
2. Xatena to bring blockchain based supply chain for medical devices (2020). https://www.startupticker.ch/en/news/january-2020/xatena-to-bring-blockchain-based-supply-chain-for-medical-devices. Accessed 1 March 2021
3. Novikova K (2019) Top 5 blockchain projects in healthcare. Latest examples of blockchain projects in healthcare. https://digiforest.io/en/blog/blockchain-examples-in-healthcare
4. Blockchains: The great chain of being sure about things. The Economist. 31 October 2015. Archived from the original on 3 July 2016. https://web.archive.org/web/20160703000844, http://www.economist.com/news/briefing/21677221-technology-behind-bitcoin-lets-people-who-do-not-know-or-trust-each-other-build-dependable. Accessed 4 March 2021
5. Narayanan A, Bonneau J, Felten E, Miller A, Goldfeder S (2016) Bitcoin and cryptocurrency technologies: a comprehensive introduction. Princeton University Press
6. Krawiec R. Blockchain: Opportunities for Health Care. Deloitte US. 2016. URL: https://www2.deloitte.com/content/dam/Deloitte/us/Documents/public-sector/us-blockchain-opportunities-for-health-care.pdf. Accessed 8 March 2021
7. Angraal S, Krumholz IIM, Schulz WL (2017) Blockchain technology: applications in health care. Circul Cardiovascular Qual Outcomes 10(9):e003800
8. Kramer DB, Fu K (2017) Cybersecurity concerns and medical devices: lessons from a pacemaker advisory. JAMA 318(21):2077–2078
9. O'Brien G, Edwards S, Littlefield K, McNab N, Wang S, Zheng K, Securing wireless infusion pumps. NIST Special Publication. 1800:8B
10. Gibson A, Thamilarasu G (2020) Protect your pacemaker: blockchain based authentication and consented authorization for implanted medical devices. Procedia Comput Sci. 171:847–856
11. Friedman S (2018) FDA builds blockchain-based health data sharing platform. https://gcn.com/articles/2018/06/22/fda-blockchain-chr-sharing.aspx. Accessed 5 March 2021
12. Alexander A, McGill M, Tarasova A, Ferreira C, Zurkiya D (2019) Scanning the future of medical imaging. J Amer College Radiol 16(4, Part A):501–7
13. Ahmed M, Pathan ASK (2020) Blockchain: can it be trusted? Computer 53(4):31–35
14. Srivastava G, Crichigno J, Dhar S (eds) A light and secure healthcare blockchain for iot medical devices. 2019 IEEE Canadian conference of electrical and computer engineering (CCECE). IEEE
15. Garg N, Wazid M, Das AK, Singh DP, Rodrigues JJPC, Park Y (2020) BAKMP-IoMT: design of blockchain enabled authenticated key management protocol for internet of medical things deployment. IEEE Access. 8:95956–95977
16. Ellouze F, Fersi G, Jmaiel M (eds) (2020) Blockchain for internet of medical things: a technical review. International conference on smart homes and health telematics. Springer
17. Cyran MA (2018) Blockchain as a foundation for sharing healthcare data. Blockchain Healthcare Today 1:1–6
18. Healthcare Data Breach Statistics (2021) HIPAA J. https://www.hipaajournal.com/healthcare-data-breach-statistics. Accessed 5 March 2021
19. Wince R (2018) real world use cases of blockchain for medical devices. https://www.medtechintelligence.com/feature_article/real-world-use-cases-of-blockchain-for-medical-devices. Accessed 5 March 2021
20. Goel U, Ruhl R, Zavarsky P (2019) using healthcare authority and patient blockchains to develop a tamperproof record tracking system.https://doi.org/10.1109/BigDataSecurity-HPSC-IDS.2019.00016
21. Li P, Nelson SD, Malin BA, Chen Y (2019) DMMS: a decentralized blockchain ledger for the management of medication histories. Blockchain Healthcare Today 2

22. Wamba SF, Anand A, Carter L (2013) A literature review of RFID-enabled healthcare applications and issues. Int J Inf Manage 33(5):875–891
23. Bell L, Buchanan WJ, Cameron J, Lo O (2019) Applications of blockchain within healthcare. Blockchain Healthcare Today1(8).
24. IBM Institute for Business Value. Healthcare rallies for blockchains (2016). https://www.ibm.com/downloads/cas/BBRQK3WY. Accessed 15 April 2021
25. Xu X, Lu Q, Liu Y, Zhu L, Yao H, Vasilakos AV (2019) Designing blockchain-based applications a case study for imported product traceability. Futur Gener Comput Syst 1 (92):399–406
26. Xia X et al (2019) Design of traceability system for medical devices based on blockchain. J Phys Conf Ser 1314,012067
27. Huh S, Cho S, Kim S (2017) Managing IoT devices using blockchain platform. In: 2017 19th international conference on advanced communication technology (ICACT) 2017 Feb 19. IEEE, pp. 464–467
28. Hewa T, Ylianttila M, Liyanage M (2020) Survey on blockchain based smart contracts: applications, opportunities and challenges. J Network Comput Appl 177
29. Trust & Automation Between Companies. Chronicled (2019). https://www.chronicled.com. Accessed 3 March 2021
30. Clauson KA, Breeden EA, Davidson C, Mackey TK (2018) Leveraging blockchain technology to enhance supply chain management in healthcare: an exploration of challenges and opportunities in the health supply chain. Blockchain Healthcare Today. 1(3):1–12
31. Brøgger-Mikkelsen M, Ali Z, Zibert JR, Andersen AD, Thomsen SF (2020) Online patient recruitment in clinical trials: systematic review and meta-analysis. J Med Internet Res 22(11): e22179. https://doi.org/10.2196/22179
32. Hasan O, Brunie L, Bertino E (2020) Privacy preserving reputation systems based on blockchain and other cryptographic building blocks: a survey: University of Lyon; INSA-Lyon; CNRS-LIRIS-UMR5205
33. Marco I, Lakhani KR (2017) The truth about blockchain. Harv Bus Rev 95(1):118–127
34. Dunn J (2019) IoT in healthcare: blockchain use cases and why they matter. https://espeoblockchain.com/blog/iot-in-healthcare. Accessed 4 March 2021
35. Pane J, Verhamme KMC, Shrum L, Rebollo I, Sturkenboom MCJM (2020) Blockchain technology applications to postmarket surveillance of medical devices. Expert Rev Med Devices 17(10):1123–1132
36. Software as a Medical Device (SAMD): Clinical Evaluation. Guidance for industry and food and drug administration staff (2017). https://www.fda.gov/regulatory-information/search-fda-guidance-documents/software-medical-device-samd-clinical-evaluation. Accessed 4 March 2021
37. Clinical Decision Support Software. Draft guidance for industry and food and drug administration staff (2019). https://www.fda.gov/regulatory-information/search-fda-guidance-documents/clinical-decision-support-software. Accessed 4 March 2021
38. Dimitrov DV (2019) Blockchain applications for healthcare data management. Healthc Inform Res 25(1):51–56
39. Bitcoin Daily Transactions (2021). https://charts.bitcoin.com/bch/chart/daily-transactions#5ma4. Accessed 3 March 2021
40. Gross MS, Miller Jr RC (2019) Ethical implementation of the learning healthcare system with blockchain technology. Blockchain Healthcare Today Forthcoming
41. Bell L, Buchanan WJ, Cameron J, Lo O (2018) Applications of blockchain within healthcare. Blockchain Healthcare Today 1(8)
42. Gaynor M, Tuttle-Newhall J, Parker J, Patel A, Tang C (2020) Adoption of blockchain in health care. J Med Internet Res 22(9):e17423

Application of Blockchain Technology in Healthcare Supply Chains

14

Venkataramanaiah Saddikuti, Sagar Galwankar, and S. V. Akilesh Sai

The supply chain stuff is really tricky.

—Elon Musk, CEO of Tesla and SpaceX

Abstract

Blockchain Technology (BCT) has been applied across many fields including healthcare. It has gained popularity due to its inherent advantages like real time, traceability, decentralisation, and high levels of security. BCT in healthcare has been applied in different areas like hospital services, pharmaceutical industry, clinical diagnostics, billing and claims, end user services etc. In this chapter we present Blockchain technology framework and its applications in healthcare supply chains along with challenges and opportunities. We also highlight important insights and conclusions.

Keyword

Blockchain · Healthcare · Supply chain · Traceability · Security

V. Saddikuti (✉)
Indian Institute of Management Lucknow, Lucknow, India
e-mail: svenkat@iiml.ac.in

S. Galwankar
Director for Research in Emergency Medicine, Florida State University,
Sarasota Memorial Hospital, Florida, USA

S. V. Akilesh Sai
Sapienza University, Rome, Italy

Introduction to Blockchain Technology

Blockchain is a distributed system and based on cryptographic techniques and helps in connected transactions. The data is located in a network of personal computers called nodes where there is no central entity controlling the data. According to Nakamoto [21], Blockchain is defined as a "decentralised, distributed, immutable ledger which is used to securely record transactions across many computers in a peer-to-peer network without the need of third party". In Blockchain all data is shared publicly although the contents of each data are only accessible to those with permission. Blockchain technology enhances data safety, reliability, integrity, transparency and reduces transaction cost [4, 13, 23]. Conventional centralized networks store data in a central server so that only a single central institution has access to the information. Blockchain technology provides platform for creating and distributing the ledger of a transaction to several computers linked to networks [1]. In contrast, Blockchain-based distribution networks assign an account that contain distributable data to each user. In Blockchain networks, hacking is difficult because anyone who wishes to modify the stored data will have to simultaneously hack into a vast number of user accounts [18]. Blockchain technology works on five principles (i) distributed database, (ii) peer-to-peer transmission, (iii) Transparency of transactions, (iv) irreversibility of records and (v) computational logic

Gregory and Savic [8] Figure 14.1 shows the elements and working mechanism of Blockchain Technology [24]. These elements can be classified broadly into technology (Information and communication technology), people (users/stakeholders) and processes (transaction validation, verification and execution) related and their interconnectedness.

We have used the key word search to find relevant literature on Blockchain Technology and its applications in healthcare from the databases like EBSCO, Google Scholar, internet sources, various journals and industry reports, review of academic research on Blockchain technology and healthcare. This chapter is organised into five sections. Blockchain Technology framework is given in section "Blockchain Technology Framework and Types". Section three focus on applications of BCT in healthcare supply chains, various challenges and opportunities of BCT in healthcare in section four followed by insights and conclusions in section five.

Blockchain Technology Framework and Types

Blockchain technology (BCT) has been adopted by many companies and governments around the world. BCT uses combination of data and transactions which are registered in a distributed network. Blockchain technology was proposed by Nakamoto [21] through the use of cryptocurrencies like Bitcoin. BCT operates as a peer-to-peer network without a central authority/ third party. Figure 14.2 shows the structure of Blockchain technology. The structure of BCT ensures that the system is

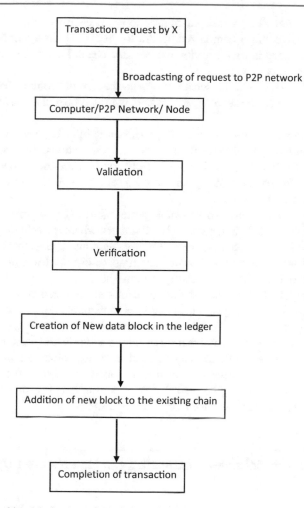

Fig. 14.1 Working Mechanism of Blockchain Technology

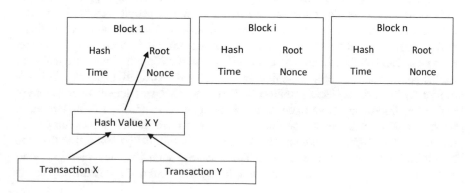

Fig. 14.2 Typical Blockchain Structure

open to those who like to make a transaction. This ensures safer, anonymous, persistent, traceable and decentralized access to users [21]. An identification code ("hash"), is contained in each addition made to the chain. Data can be tracked with a higher level of accuracy.

There are four types of Blockchain networks that are in use in different sectors. These include public, private, consortium and hybrid Blockchains [25].

- **Public Blockchains** has no special type of restriction. Anyone on internet can connect with this type of network and can send transactions. The user can act as a key validator. Public Blockchains generally consider economic incentive-based mechanisms for securing the system through effective utilization of the special type of consensus algorithm.
- **Private Blockchains** are also known as permissioned (i.e., a person needs to be invited by the Blockchain network administrator), where the role of participation and validator is very much restricted. Organization and applications that require handling of sensitive data and record-keeping mainly opt for a private permissioned approach for Blockchain infrastructure access.
- **Consortium Blockchains** are referred as semi-decentralized Blockchain, where multiple organizations together take decision to facilitate the Blockchain service provisioning to the users. Permissioned approach is fitted over the users
- **Hybrid Blockchains** is a combination of public and private Blockchain network facilities. Such type of Blockchain is used in reality when conglomeration of public and private data access is seamlessly incorporated over the user. In this Blockchain, the users may be provided with permissioned or free access based on specific implications as needed by the application.

Application of Blockchain Technology in Healthcare Supply Chains

Innovations in healthcare industry primarily aimed at improving quality of life, life expectancy, treatment options and cost efficiency and patient safety. Artificial Intelligence (AI) and Machine Learning (ML) approaches are driving the huge cost reductions and early detection of health status of the people across the world. Blockchain technology has been applied in diverse fields such as finance, distribution, logistics, public services, arts, healthcare etc. [18]. According to market report on Blockchain technology in healthcare sector (Supply chain, clinical data exchange, claims and billing, end user services) is expected to reach US\$ 829 million by 2023 from US\$ 54 million in 2018 [19]. Of late, Blockchain technology has gained importance from many areas including medicine [3, 7, 18]. In particular, the use of Blockchain technology in the transfer of medical data allows the patient rather than the hospital to own medical data. As a result, the patient rather than the hospital has control over medical data. This enables patients to conveniently submit a complete set of medical data to any hospital upon transfer, and it helps physicians gain a better understanding of patients based on the submitted data and plan suitable treatments. Application of BCT can help in reducing the healthcare costs by avoiding redundant medical examinations, better use of medicines and diagnostics, efficient billing and processing etc. It helps in reducing the risk of potential disclosure of patient medical information [7]. Application of Blockchain in healthcare supply chains ensures secured access to medical data of patients and other stakeholders like insurance companies, hospitals, doctors etc. [26]. COVID-19 pandemic is a big opportunity for many organisations to go for Blockchain technology in mitigating and managing the crisis [10]. These advantages of Blockchain technology are expected to have a positive influence on clinicians and patients.

Healthcare sector is facing major issues like complex and fragmented supply chains (SCs), inefficient data management, insecure data sharing, data privacy challenge, drug counterfeiting, etc. According to WHO [30] study, more than 100,000 people die in Africa due to counterfeit drugs and improper dosing. Jayaraman et al. [12] noted that packaging errors and lack product registry are the major reasons for supply chain disruptions. These issues in healthcare are the major reasons for slower treatments, poorer health management and public-backlash. These can be addressed by enhancing the data management capabilities using Blockchain technology. Blockchain can be used to improve patient outcomes, lower costs, enhance compliance and ensure security, transparency and better use of healthcare data [20]. The information can be kept safe and secure in Blockchains and access could be provided to all related parties. The application of Blockchain is growing very rapidly in many areas of healthcare. These include, neuroscience, electronic health records (EHR)/ electronic medical records (EMR), genomics medicine, biomedicine, clinical trials, vaccine supply and traceability, Internet of Things (IoT), pharma industry, managing drug recalls, drug counterfeiting [11, 22]. Tseng et al. [29] to address double spending and counterfeiting problems associated with pharma supply chain. Blockchain technology has been applied for maintaining data integrity, access and management of health records in the biomedical domain [6]. Blockchains are used to solve the worldwide trade of counterfeit medicines [17]. Blockchain are also used for managing blood from corruption and adulteration and to ensure visibility of the entire blood supply chain [15], monitoring temperature and other parameters of sensitive drugs [5]. Blockchain based smart contracts are used in protecting intellectual property rights. Blockchain is also facilitating better in academic medicine in the areas like evidence-based medicine, performance evaluation of students and teachers [28]. Major areas of application of Blockchain Technology in healthcare supply chain include.

- Electronic medical records
- Remote patient monitoring
- Smart contracts with vendors
- Drug traceability

- Product recalls and reverse logistics
- Managing product shortages and obsolescence
- Turnaround time management
- Efficient inventory management
- Clinical trials and precision medicine
- Preventive maintenance and tracking of medical equipment and devices
- Research and Development in medical and pharmaceutical sector
- Health Insurance claims and bills processing
- Medical staff credentials verification
- Public health supply chains for disaster and emergency mitigation and management
- Elimination of errors, frauds/counterfeits in the healthcare system
- Identification of bottlenecks and process improvement
- Overall cost reduction and quality improvement
- Improved Patient safety and trust
- Prevention of informal practices in the health systems

Application of BCT in healthcare supply chains help in improving or replacing slow manual processes, strengthening traceability, reducing supply chain IT transaction costs. It helps in real time monitoring of supply chains and enhances the resilience. It helps in design of value driven solution design, improves business process capability and seamless integration with other functions of the organisation. More specifically, in case of clinical supply chains it helps in waste management, quality of clinical trials, temperature deviations across supply chains and personalisation of treatment protocols etc. [14]. Application of BCT in healthcare systems help in improving the efficiency of care delivery and patient safety. Smart contracts with vendors will contribute in improved responsiveness, leadtime reduction, transaction costs reduction, increased visibility and more trust, security and transparency across the supply chain. Blockchain technology can help in quick response during public health emergencies and product recalls [16].

Challenges and Opportunities for Adoption of Blockchain in Healthcare Supply Chains

Blockchain technology also faces several challenges such as governance, organisational, integration, ethical issues, security, privacy, latency and throughput, Blockchain size, computing power, storage requirements, scalability, interoperability and standardisation etc. Incidences of healthcare data breaches, threat of counterfeit drugs, reluctance to data disclosures, lack of common standards etc. are major challenges for large scale adoption of BCT in healthcare. Ben Fekih and Lahami [26] and Jayaraman et al. [11] have identified the following major challenges in the application of Blockchain Technologies in healthcare

- **Interoperability**: EMR systems do not address interoperability and as a result, manual inspection and mapping of predefined ontologies from medical and health data experts are required. This issue can be addressed by developing standards based on BCT
- **Clinical malpractice** cannot be controlled
- **Scalability** is a big challenge due to high volume of medical data which cannot be stored on the Blockchain
- **Latency** due to speed of transactions' processing
- **Immutability** and self-execution of code, since smart contracts could become vulnerable to hackers.
- **Generating standards-** there are no comprehensive standards for Supply chains.
- **Data accuracy-** in case of supply chains there are many steps involved and collection and monitoring of big data sets is a costly affair
- Payment/funding of blockchain technology is still not clear.

Apart from the above, social challenge like cultural issues is a major concerned. Privacy and data protection is one of the major challenges and needs suitable regulations and national and international level. Lack of standards for product identifiers across supply chain is concerned at global level. Fragmented data and information and mixed product lots etc.

Application of Blockchain technology in healthcare has many advantages which is similar to that of internet, mobile phones etc. It can help in reducing the costs as well as time along the continuum of healthcare delivery and improve transparency and patient safety. Developing standards for data storage and handling will be a great opportunity for many organisations including healthcare start-ups [2, 9, 27].

Insights and Conclusions

Application of Blockchain Technology in healthcare is revolutionising the way healthcare is delivered. It is facilitating better in improving patient safety and reducing supply chain costs. Blockchain application in healthcare is reforming traditional healthcare towards a reliable and effective diagnosis and treatment. Blockchain in healthcare benefit almost all stakeholders including patients, medical practitioners, insurance providers, R & D organisations, pharmaceutical companies, diagnostic service providers, medical equipment and device manufacturers and supply chain stakeholders and government agencies. BCT in healthcare ensures security and privacy of the medical records and patient safety. COVID-19 pandemic also adding to the speed of adoption of Blockchain in healthcare supply chains. It helps in improving traceability, obsolescence, shortages, pilferage, transparency etc. Based on various studies, it shows that medical care is moving towards personalised and secured healthcare delivery in real time.

However, Blockchain in healthcare is not free from various challenges. These challenges include fragmented supply chains, data privacy, lack of data standards and regulations, data sharing and trust among the supply chain stakeholders. These challenges need to be addressed at industry level for fast and large-scale implementation. Further studies can focus on developing data standards and regulations for large scale implementation at industry level.

References

1. Alicke K, Davies A, Leopoldseder M, Nemyer A (2017) Blockchain technology for supply chains-A must or a maybe? McKinsey
2. Bahga A, Madisetti V (2016) Blockchain platform for industrial internet of things. J Softw Eng Appl 9:533–546. https://doi.org/10.4236/jsea.2016.910036
3. Casino F, Dasaklis TK, Patsakis C (2019) a systematic literature review of blockchain based applications: current, classification and open issues. Telematics Informat, 55–81.
4. Chang MC, Hau YS, Park JC, Lee JM (2019) The application of Blockchain technology in stroke rehabilitation. Amer J Phys Med Rehab 98(7):e74 PMID: 30516553
5. Clark B, Burstall R (2018) Blockchain, IP and the pharma industry—how distributed ledger technologies can help secure the pharma supply chain. J Intellectual Property Law Pract 13 (7):531–533
6. Drosatos G, Kaldoudi F (2019) Blockchain applications in the biomedical domain: a scoping review. Comput Struct Biotechnol J 17:229–240
7. El-Gazzar R, Stendal K (2020) Blockchain in healthcare: hope or Hype. J Med Int Res
8. Gregory RW, Savic B (2019) Blockchain for managers. IESE Bus School
9. Haq I, Esuka OM (2018) Blockchain technology in pharmaceutical industry to prevent counterfeit drugs. Int J Comput Appl 180(25):8–12. https://doi.org/10.5120/ijca2018916579
10. Hoek RV, Lacity M (2020) How the Pandemic is pushing Blockchain forward. Harv Bus Rev
11. Jayaraman R, Salah K, King N (2019) Improving opportunities in healthcare supply chain processes via the internet of things & blockchain technology. Int J Healthcare Inform Syst Inform 14(2):49–65. https://doi.org/10.4018/IJHISI.2019040104
12. Jayaraman R, AlHammadi F, Simsekler MCE (2018) Managing product recalls in healthcare supply chain. In: Proceedings of the 2018 IEEE international conference on industrial engineering and engineering management (IEEM), Bangkok, Thailand, 16–19 December 2018; pp 293–297
13. Jo BW, Khan RMA, Lee YS (2018) Hybrid Blockchain and internet-of-things network for underground structure health monitoring. Sensors (Basel) 18(12). PMID: 30518124
14. Kachwala M, Kilgore C, KInscher K, Talwar V (2021) Clinical supply chains: how to boost excellence and innovation. McKinsey
15. Kim HM, Laskowski M (2018) toward an ontology-driven blockchain design for supply-chain provenance. Intell Syst Account Financ Manag 25(1):18–27
16. Lim KM, Li Y, Wang C, Tseng ML (2021) A literature review of blockchain technology applications in supply chains: a comprehensive analysis of themes, methodologies and industries. Comput Indus Eng 154. https://doi.org/10.1016/j.cie.2021.107133
17. Mackey TK , Nayyar G (2017) A review of existing and emerging digital technologies to combat the global trade in fake medicines. Expert Opinion Drug Safety 16(11). https://doi.org/10.1080/14740338.2017.1313227
18. Mackey TK, Kuo TT, Gummadi B, Clauson KA, Church G, Grishin D, Obbad K, Barkovich R, Palombini M (2019) 'Fit-for-purpose?'—challenges and opportunities for applications of Blockchain technology in the future of healthcare. BMC Med 17(1):68 PMID: 30914045

19. Markets and Markets (2018) Blockchain technology in healthcare market, blockchain technology in healthcare market size, share and Trends forecast to 2023 by application, End User | COVID-19 Impact Analysis | MarketsandMarkets™

20. Mattke J, Maier C, HundA., Weitzel T (2019) How an enterprise blockchain application in the U.S. pharmaceuticals supply chain is saving lives. MIS Quart Executive 18(4):245–261

21. Nakamoto S (2008) Bitcoin: a peer-to-peer electronic cash system. https://bitcoin.org/bitcoin.pdf

22. Padmavati U, Rajagopalan N (2019) A research on impact of blockchain in healthcare. Int J Innov Technol Exploring. Eng 8(9):35–40

23. Park JS, Youn TY, Kim HB, Rhee KH, Shin SU (2018) Smart contract-based review system for an IoT data marketplace. Sensors (Basel) 18(10). PMID: 30360413

24. PwC (2018) Making sense of bitcoin, cryptocurrency and Blockchain. https://www.pwc.com/us/en/industries/financial-services/fintech/bitcoin-blockchain-cryptocurrency.html

25. Ray PP, Dash D, Salah K, Kumar N (2021) Blockchain for IoT-based healthcare: background, consensus, platforms, and use cases. IEEE Syst J 15(1):85–94

26. Rim Ben Fekih R, Mariam Lahami M (2020) application of blockchain technology in healthcare: a comprehensive study in ICOST 2020, pp 268–276. https://doi.org/10.1007/978-3-030-51517-1_23

27. Srivastava SC, Shainesh G (2015) Bridging the service divide through digitally enabled service innovations: evidence from Indian Healthcare service providers. MIS Q 39(1):245–267

28. Stawicki SP, Firstenberg MS, Papadimos TJ (2018) What's new in academic medicine? Blockchain technology in health-care: Bigger, better, fairer, faster, and leaner. Int J Acad Med 4:1–11

29. Tseng J-H, Liao Y-C, Chong B, Liao S-W (2018) Governance on the drug supply chain via gcoin Blockchain. Int J Environ Res Public Health 15(6):1055

30. WHO (2017) WHO global surveillance and monitoring system for substandard and falsified medical products. World Health Organisation: Geneva, Switzerland

The Use of Blockchain in Fighting Medical Misinformation: A Concept Paper

15

Stanislaw P. Stawicki, Michael S. Firstenberg, and Thomas J. Papadimos

> *Misinformation destroys trust. When you destroy trust, you destroy the bonds that hold society together.*
>
> —Laurence Overmire

Abstract

The security, anonymity, speed, and accessibility of blockchain technology has the potential to help the medical scientific community create a dynamic consensus protocol that can rapidly adapt to today's changing social, scientific, and political landscape. Unchecked medical misinformation has been a serious problem during the coronavirus disease 2019 (COVID-19) pandemic and has hindered the implementation of effective medical and public health measures. Blockchain technology will facilitate a scientific consensus among members of the scientific community regarding which scientific claims constitute a scientific

S. P. Stawicki (✉)
Department of Research and Innovation, St. Luke's University Health Network, Bethlehem, PA 18015, USA
e-mail: stawicki.ace@gmail.com

M. S. Firstenberg
Director of Research and Special Projects, William Novick Global Cardiac Alliance, Memphis, TN, USA
e-mail: msfirst@gmail.com

T. J. Papadimos
Department of Anesthesiology, The Ohio State University Wexner Medical Center, Columbus, OH 43210, USA
e-mail: tjpapadimos@gmail.com

fact, and lead to public transparency of such discourses now and in future exigencies. Therein mitigating the spread of unchecked medical misinformation that can result in both serious and unpredictable consequences to a society.

Keywords

Blockchain · Censorship · Disinformation · Information management · Misinformation · Oversight · Public harm · Social media · Source credibility

Introduction

Medical misinformation (MEMI) occurs when individuals propagate health-related claims as "medical fact," without proper scientific verification, falsely asserting that the content being communicated is indeed true [1–3]. Lack of rigorous scientific vetting of medical information that is shared across a broad range of modern media platforms results in a potentially dangerous *status quo* [4–6]. Despite being difficult to quantify, actual harm resulting from MEMI can be very significant and may affect multiple segments of society (e.g., economic, health, social, etc.) [7–11].

Consequences of unchecked MEMI can be serious and unpredictable, often resulting in unreasonable fear and anxiety among a populace [12]. The current coronavirus disease 2019 (COVID-19) pandemic does not represent the first time in history where MEMI was widespread; however, it does represent perhaps the most widespread and best documented instance(s) of MEMI in history [13, 14]. Throughout centuries, irrational fears drove humans to erroneously assign blame, create unacceptable shame, resort to ineffective treatments, and to recommend outright harmful management approaches when facing various public health threats [15–18].

What is Scientific Consensus?

Medical misinformation as a concept is closely related to the currently utilized mechanisms of reaching scientific consensus. More specifically, those who initiate and propagate MEMI often utilize opinions and data that substantially deviate from the generally accepted consensus view [5, 11]. Although leveraging such "dissenting views" to generate new hypotheses and further scientific discord is generally accepted, and even encouraged to some degree, problems tend to arise when non-experts begin to propagate MEMI based on "individual beliefs" or other "secondary" factors (e.g., "political orientation" or "group membership") [19–23].

Scientific consensus (SC) refers to an agreement among scientific community members about which scientific claims (e.g., statements proposing an explanation about an empirical phenomenon) constitute a scientific fact (a true, proven claim) [22–24]. In this chapter, we propose the development of a distributed mechanism for the determination of an urgently needed medical SC (MSC) to curb the escalating phenomenon of MEMI associated with the unchecked and exponential growth of Internet-based media platforms. Further, it is proposed that blockchain technology (BCT)-based MSC verification can be implemented and fill the critically needed scientific consensus-building gap that currently exists. Moreover, this can be accomplished in a way that is constructive and minimally restrictive from the standpoint of preserving scientific freedom and reduce the potential harm resulting from the "unchecked dissemination" of MEMI across contemporary media platforms (both conventional and non-conventional "social media" outlets).

Will Consensus Mechanisms be Effective in Curtailing Medical Misinformation?

To reach MSC, the medical scientific community's members employ their collective scientific training, experience, and knowledge to verify claims through the use of the scientific method. Although not perfect by any means, this process involves a comprehensive and objective assessment of the peer-reviewed literature, and is very transparent (e.g., each peer-reviewed item is clearly labeled as such, and non-peer-reviewed items are flagged accordingly) [25–27]. With the accumulation of sufficient research intended to verify a particular claim, the scientific community can increase the cumulative probability that any particular claim is indeed true (or untrue). In a way, one might reframe the above by stating that when each member of the scientific community is "more than 50% certain" of the claim's validity, then a consensus (at least a preliminary one) regarding the validity of the claim has been reached. Over time, given the presence of consistently increasing degrees of probability, one can also begin to interpret a particular claim as a "scientific fact" [28, 29]. Of great importance, and to be determined at a later time, is the decision regarding which members of the scientific community are eligible to determine a particular claim's validity, and what percentage of that suitable/qualified expert group would be required to cause a "scientific claim" to gradually become a "scientific fact" (or alternatively, to become "disproven"). Regardless of the above considerations, without MSC, a claim remains only a "claim" and does not become admitted into the realm of "facts" [30–32].

Another important consideration in this context is the presence of various mechanisms that exist primarily to "disprove" certain points of view. Although such mechanisms are very important in the overall search for scientific truth, they can also be misused by those who simply are trying to make a point without regard for its merits/validity [33, 34]. True dangers of this particular approach become evident when different pseudo-scientific arguments enter the mainstream, either as economic or political points of discord [35, 36]. The current coronavirus disease 2019 (COVID-19) pandemic is unfortunately a leading example of the misuse and misinterpretation of scientific facts toward non-scientific (and often harmful) ends [37, 38]. Other examples of similar misuse were described by Plaza, et al., and include the case of the autism-vaccine controversy and the activities of the fluoride action network [5]. In summary, although it is important to begin constructing robust processes to address the above-mentioned issues and challenges, much remains to be "agreed upon"—including the optimal "level of agreement." Specifically, is "greater than 50%" sufficient? Or do we need stricter guidelines and thresholds?

How Good Intentions Lead to Harm: Fact Versus Belief

Medical misinformation usually does not begin as a malicious endeavor. In fact, the most common mode of the propagation of MEMI is through well-meant actions of those who are deeply passionate about a particular cause [5]. This, in itself, is a potentially positive development in that MEMI may be correctable in its earliest phases, primarily via the introduction of appropriate content experts who may be able to re-introduce scientific balance into an otherwise unbalanced discourse. Educational efforts aimed at increasing awareness of MEMI within the general population constitute an important adjunctive measure. If an early intervention does not take place, MEMI can enter the phase of exponential dissemination. Once widely disseminated, MEMI may be very difficult to rectify (especially considering that high-profile challenges to established lines of thinking often generate significant interest and reporting in both the conventional journalistic media and the less rigorously reviewed social media outlets [often turning the more controversial, outlandish, or dramatic highlights and potentially incorrectly so into brief sound bites or tweets]) [39, 40]. Such developments may render the scientific community effectively powerless to restore the content back into the realm of MSC-building.

In one well established example, the very public controversy regarding the alleged relationship between the measles, mumps, and rubella (MMR) vaccination and the increasing incidence of autism, demonstrates how pervasive MEMI can become once "out in the open" [41, 42]. In this particular instance, a now-retracted high-profile publication in the journal *Lancet*, was found to contain critical methodological errors that essentially invalidate any conclusion of the paper exploring the link between MMR vaccine and autism [5, 43]. Yet despite the above shortcomings of the original study, the prevalence of misguided beliefs regarding the issue was found to be much greater among areas that experienced greater media attention to the issue [43, 44]. This highlights a unique set of challenges that is often faced by scientific authorities engaged in rectifying the damage from MEMI—the combination of "science turned into belief" and the prevalence of "misguided believers" who are unwilling to consider the alternative explanation(s) and/or arguments [45, 46].

In the case of MMR vaccination, the real-world consequences were (and in certain areas continue to be) truly devastating, with parents worldwide deciding to stop vaccinating their children. In the United Kingdom, the MMR vaccination rate dropped from 92% in 1996 to 85% in 2002. In the United States, there was a noticeable drop in MMR vaccination rate between 1996 and 2002. The decrease in the vaccination rates of children likely contributed to the 2014–2015 measles outbreak in the United States, where an estimated 125 people contracted the disease, as well as the more recent, much larger outbreak of 2018–2019 [47–50]. The largest spike of measles in decades, prompted the Centers for Disease Control and Prevention to release the press statement, "U. S. measles cases in first five months of 2019 surpass total cases per year for past 25 years," demonstrating the long-lasting repercussions and residual damage of MEMI [51–53].

Providing Balance: The Case of *Helicobacter Pylori*:

Not all claims made by well-established "mainstream" scientific community prevail in the long-term. Yet the damage done to individual scientists' reputations for standing up to the establishment may be severe and long-lasting, demonstrating the opposite of the intended effect of the scientific process. One powerful example of such a case is the 1955 scientific consensus that bacteria were not the cause of peptic ulcers [5, 54, 55]. Because of the widespread acceptance of this consensus, most members of the medical scientific community remained skeptical of Dr. Robin Warren and Dr. Barry Marshall's research which argued that *Helicobacter pylori* was the cause of peptic ulcers [56, 57]. Being faced by an overwhelming opposing majority, both the physician-scientists experienced both stigma and prejudice because of their research. Fortunately, they persisted and, over the course of 30 years, collected a substantial amount of evidence consistently proving their theory. In the early 1980s, the scientific community finally committed to a new MSC, the one in which peptic ulcers were determined to be caused *by H. pylori* [58, 59]. Within the context of our chapter, this particular example demonstrates how a group of determined scientists were able to sway the "opposing majority" by consistently and accurately utilizing scientific experiments (and ultimately facts) to convince—rather than force—others that a particular point of view is indeed a correct one. Moreover, two key differences between this particular example and those outlined in the previous sections, is that the current scenario was largely "debated and settled" within the scientific community and that there was no significant public, political, or social media involvement in the matter. Consequently, the latter statement supports the position that deleterious effect(s) of social media platforms do indeed exist as it pertains to the introduction of unfair biases into what should be primarily scientific discourse.

Movement Toward Potential Solutions

All of the above examples emphasize the importance of the need for an impartial, high-integrity system that is not subject to any economic or political influences, while at the same time providing ample and appropriate content expertise in pertinent subject areas. It is unlikely that such system will be attainable in the near future. However, some simple measures can ensure that bias and undue influences are minimized. For example, members of the scientific community must continue to be vigilant when conducting the peer-review process, especially when highly controversial topics and findings have the potential of introducing public health dangers through the propagation of MEMI across various social media channels.

Medical institutions, public organizations, and scientific journals must ensure that their members strictly abide by the established MSC processes. Complacency has the potential to result in MEMI because of poorly filtered information now being allowed to interface directly with both established social media and mainstream media data "intake" mechanisms. Thus, an environment without proper checks and balances may end up in the publication and subsequent misinterpretation of critical information in some of the most prestigious medical journals in the world [5]. The number of "layers of review" may decrease the probability of poorly conducted peer review, but still does not guarantee that the final product will be accurate, unbiased, and scientifically sound. Finally, the duration of post-publication "exposure" appears to correlate with how deeply ingrained MEMI becomes within the general population (e.g., the anti-vaccine movement) [5].

The cumulative "lessons learned" from the examples discussed herein provide a good conceptual starting point for strengthening the overall scientific process, beginning with the planning phase and extending well into the post-publication information dissemination phase. Within the context of the current chapter and the current book, one solution is to explore potential applications of blockchain technology (BCT). This is because its decentralized consensus methodology is inherently suitable to facilitate other types of consensus building [60, 61]. In brief, BCT is a computationally governed public ledger that permanently records all transactions in a chain of interlinked data packets (also known as, "blocks") [62]. As such, the blockchain utilizes a consensus mechanism that verifies and adds new transactions to the chain of preceding blocks, all based on the ability of the participating actors to "agree on validity" of the new block as the "next in line" for inclusion. Such consensus mechanism ensures integrity and consistency across geographically distributed, independently operated nodes. More detailed/technical discussions of this process can be found in earlier chapters of this book.

Blockchain and Scientific Consensus: From Inception to Post-Publication

In the jargon of BCT, "distributed nodes" are decentralized junctions that allow for the node operators to use the blockchain to process, transmit, or receive specified transactions. Node operators (e.g., people or institutions) are the active participants of the blockchain. Collectively, all the nodes within the network help facilitate the computational operation(s) of the blockchain through simple yet very powerful consensus mechanism(s). Finally, the node operators have the ability to participate in a "voting system" to agree upon the way the consensus mechanism will manage the blockchain. A blockchain-based MSC model presents certain challenges that must be carefully fleshed out, such as who and what authority will define who the members of the scientific community and node operators are, and what the respective qualifying criteria will be. It is important to a void a strictly demo-cratic format (e.g., the largest number of opinions decides), as that is not necessarily synonymous with the presence of factual and/or scientific correctness [5, 62].

It is also critically important to recognize that not all claims contrary to the prevailing SCS/MSC eventually turn out to be false. History is replete with erro-neous ideas that were subsequently wholly and completely accepted by the scien-tific community (e.g., egocentricity versus heliocentricity) at some point in time. Dissenting opinions often take very long to gain momentum against the existing tide of "scientific belief" and the prevailing knowledge base. As our knowledge base continues to expand, and technology that facilitates further discoveries im-proves, we will undoubtedly make new discoveries that may contradict our pre-vious understanding of a particular subject (or some of its nuances). The scientific community must be conscientious in avoiding mechanism(s) that act as barrier(s) to the changing perspectives of medicine and science as our understanding evolves over time. Consequently, as our knowledge of a topic evolves, it is inevitable that our understanding of a particular disease and/or treatment will change as well. In this context, we must be careful that the "majority consensus" does not act as a "majority dictatorship" or a barrier to make it more difficult to change the past dogma which is believed to be true when there is a dissenting opinion or a con-trarian theoretical proposal [63–65].

There is limited research on the relationship between existing BCT capabilities/implementations and scientific consensus building. Such a relationship, however, inherently makes sense. If one views the scientists (or members of the scientific community) as the "node operators" of the blockchain, who use the ledger to transact their scientific research information, review, and verification, then BCT can be helpful in enhancing the attainment of MSC in several ways. First, imple-mentation of BCT-based MSC could help secure the process of consensus building (by making it both transparent and immutable). Second, it would make the process of MSC building more objective and less biased. Third, it would provide scientists with anonymity while also preventing specific "agendas" from overtaking the fairness of the process through random assignment and wide geographic/institutional distribution of nodes. Fourth, BCT could both encourage communication and increase the speed and quality of communication between scientists (e.g., by enabling instant and seamless aggregation of individual "expert inputs"). Finally, the availability of a decentralized consensus-building capacity may help improve the general access to robust mechanisms intended specifically for MSC creation [66, 67]. This may ultimately lower the "barriers to entry" for new scientists and those with innovative ideas but limited ability to network and/or disseminate information.

In terms of practical implementations of BCT in the area of scientific consensus building, one clear benefit of blockchain is the enhanced data security and efficiency of MSC based on the synergy between cryptographic encryption and immutability of the record. Consequently, any dishonest or malignant actors are effectively prevented from distorting or altering the recorded information, and no one without an appropriate level of permission can access either the blockchain or its contents [68, 69]. Moreover, any changes or edits within the data are permanently recorded and readily trackable. The blockchain, therefore, allows for the secure storing and sharing of research work, with full transparency, among a specific community of scientists or experts [5]. To further augment this paradigm, once scientists believe that they have arrived at MSC regarding a certain scientific claim, they can use their node operator voting rights to formally "confirm or reject" the scientific claim as a "scientific fact" or "disproven hypothesis." At the conclusion of this voting process, BCT can provide the capacity to create/add a cryptographically immutable and secure stamp to verify the interim status of the scientific research information at hand. This stamp would certify the veracity of the scientific facts.

In accordance to our previous discussion, it goes without saying that the veracity of any "scientific fact" can be revisited at future points as new data/evidence present themselves, perhaps through the introduction of required periodic re-review of scientific evidence within a specific topic area, or perhaps via a more random, spontaneous re-visiting of a particular topic by a highly dedicated scientific team(s). With all of the above considerations, one may wonder about how an essentially expert-restricted platform constitutes a benefit to the public. In fact, within the broader context of ensuring that appropriately vetted scientific knowledge (featuring both majority and minority opinions) is exposed to the public, a "read-only" output that is suitably formatted for public scrutiny (e.g., content consisting of accessible language, transparent conclusions, and other elements typical of public-facing scientific disclosure) would be made available for all non-scientists to view. Such "read-only" output would provide a balanced view that includes various dissenting opinions determined to reach sufficient threshold that would prevent the emergence of MEMI based on unrealistic scientific views.

The security of blockchain could theoretically enable an effective process of MSC creation and maintenance, at virtually all levels of the scientific process—from hypothesis generation, to data collection, to data analysis, publication of results, and even appropriate post-publication input [5]. Of importance, BCT may serve to restrict the access and distribution of preliminary research information to only those scientists who are actively involved in the research initiative and/or its peer evaluation, thus reducing the risk of uncontrolled release of invalid or unproven results. If a consensus can be established regarding the validity of particular research results, then a subsequent decision to broadcast/release these results beyond the scientific community may follow. Further, the above-mentioned blockchain-based consensus verification stamp can be used to provide an immutable certificate of authenticity, guaranteeing that the newly released scientific claims have been deemed valid by a community of qualified/appropriate experts in the field. Any information released without such an authenticity stamp should be regarded with extreme caution, and channels should be created to constructively re-direct such information back into the formal "MSC-forming" mechanism. If such re-direction can be implemented in a non-punitive, non-judgmental way, then any dissenting or "unofficial" views would then be entered into the same, highly objective process, as any other piece of scientific evidence. Of importance, we must recognize that such mechanism would go well beyond the standard "two-reviewer" evaluation process currently employed by our scientific outlets. There would be certain benefits to this, however, as any pre-vetting mechanisms would give medical journals a readily accessible (and likely more reliable) method of proceeding only with submissions that have attained community-based MSC recommendation(s). Moreover, an authenticity stamp would provide the public with an external standard by which to verify whether a specific scientific claim is likely to be valid and/or appropriately verified by experts. Finally, post-publication community-based MSC formation can be utilized to raise any "red flags" about already-published research. In other words, scientists who identify certain research reports to be methodologically flawed or internally inconsistent will have an avenue of alerting both the scientific community and the public about such concerns. The anonymity and distributed nature of this process will be crucial to its functioning, including the element of random selection of content expert reviewers, as well as the de-stigmatization of the important function of scientific whistle-blowing [70–74].

As discussed above, the scientific community has the capacity to incorrectly develop and apply MSC, and worse yet, use it to prejudge/discount legitimate efforts intended to improve the very same MSC. The result of such prejudice can lead to decades of MEMI as we have seen in the case of Dr. Warren and Dr. Marshall's experience. Blockchain can help scientific communities mitigate this problem much more effectively than any previous methodologies. In the case of *H. pylori* and its association with peptic ulcers, the provision of a way for scientists to reach alternative conclusions without the fear of being judged and ridiculed, may have saved innumerable lives during an unnecessarily long process of breaking "old habits." It is well established that people find it more difficult to unlearn or "let go" of the existing knowledge than to learn completely new facts—a problem well exemplified with the instances of MEMI outlined in our earlier discussions [75, 76].

Finally, BCT may help improve the MSC process by increasing the speed and efficiency of communication between scientists, as well as improving the scientists' access to the MSC infrastructure. Aided by the "instant nature" of Internet technology, scientists can send data to each other seamlessly, regardless of where a researcher is located geographically. All one would need to participate in the blockchain-based science consensus process is an Internet-enabled computer with a suitable software interface. With these fundamental tools, scientists can send and receive research/data from colleagues and participate in the blockchain voting process that would help verify the accuracy of scientific data and claims, as well as the validity of the corresponding results. The larger the number of scientists who work on developing a given consensus, the more efficient and robust the MSC process becomes [77–79]. As a result, the scientific community would become more effective in intercepting and/or stopping MEMI before it spreads and potentially leads to public harm.

Data Sharing and Verification

Very relevant in this particular context is the broad topic of "data sharing" [80–82] of central importance to verification/validation of scientific results is the scientific community's ability to perform independent evaluation of the underlying data, especially when considering the widespread "pressure to publish" among researchers in the competitive academic environment of today leading to an entire spectrum of problems, beginning with subtle (but still unacceptable) biases and ending with outright scientific misconduct [83–85]. Yet, despite the clear need for independent access to source information accumulated during medical research, significant barriers persist for peer reviewers tasked with determining the validity of reported results [85–87]. Within this realm, BCT may be one of the most important, and the most disruptive, influences/practical solutions to these chronic problems.

The security, anonymity, speed, and accessibility of BCT can help the medical scientific community implement a dynamic consensus protocol that can rapidly adapt to today's changing social, scientific, and political landscape. Various social media platforms have been abused by malignant actors to efficiently propagate MEMI in the recent past [33, 88, 89]. This has been further highlighted and exacerbated during the current COVID-19 pandemic [35, 36]. In 2018, a Pew Research Center study determined that only 26% of Americans can distinguish facts from opinion in the news [90, 91]. Moreover, the same authors indicated that social movements have a relatively easier time swaying the public to believe in medical misinformation. Hoping to instill positive societal change, technology companies have started to invest in BCT designed to counteract this dangerous trend. For example, in 2017, IBM (International Business Machines Corporation, Armonk, New York) filed a patent called "Blockchain for Open Scientific Research," which aims to improve scientific research efforts through BCT [5, 92]. Despite all of the recent efforts, BCT development in this important area is still in its infancy and we have likely only seen a small glimpse of its full potential. In the long run, it should be possible that social media postings of medical and/or scientific nature could undergo a continuous pre- and post-publication, blockchain-based consensus evaluation for validity, with posts deemed invalid being tagged as having "high probability" of constituting MEMI.

Conclusion

The current chapter intends to send a clear message that a "judicious application" of BCT to help construct a sustainable MSC mechanism has the potential to become one of the most powerful tools in the fight against medical misinformation and the propagation of false, misinterpreted, and/or outright harmful medical claims. Further research and development is required in this critically important and rapidly emerging area of public health—locally, nationally, and internationally. Finally, we must ensure that any expertise rendered is accompanied by a fully transparent (and verifiable) declaration of actual and/or perceived conflicts of interest. Without the latter, any system will continue to carry the flaws and burdens of today's imperfect academic/scientific reality.

References

1. Wood JL et al (2021) A pilot study of medical misinformation perceptions and training among practitioners in North Carolina (USA). INQUIRY J Health Care Organ Provision Financ 58:00469580211035742
2. Granter SR, Papke DJ (2018) Opinion: medical misinformation in the era of google: computational approaches to a pervasive problem. Proc Natl Acad Sci 115(25):6318–6321
3. Lavorgna A, Di Ronco A (2019) Medical misinformation and social harm in non-science based health practices: a multidisciplinary perspective. Routledge
4. Baker SA, Wade M, Walsh MJ (2020) Misinformation: tech companies are removing 'harmful' coronavirus content–but who decides what that means? The Conversation
5. Plaza M et al (2019) The use of distributed consensus algorithms to curtail the spread of medical misinformation. Int J Acad Med 5(2):93
6. Niemiec E (2020) COVID-19 and misinformation: Is censorship of social media a remedy to the spread of medical misinformation? EMBO Rep 21(11):e51420
7. Tran T et al (2019) An investigation of misinformation harms related to social media during humanitarian crises. In: International conference on secure knowledge management in artificial intelligence era. Springer
8. Mirza R et al (2020) Going viral: understanding medical misinformation and older adults' vaccine hesitancy. Innov Aging 4(Supplement_1):377–378
9. Pecher B et al (2020) FireAnt: claim-based medical misinformation detection and monitoring. In :Joint European conference on machine learning and knowledge discovery in databases. Springer
10. Bronstein MV, Vinogradov S (2021) Education alone is insufficient to combat online medical misinformation. EMBO Rep 22(3):e52282
11. Chrousos GP, Mentis A-FA (2020) Medical misinformation in mass and social media: an urgent call for action, especially during epidemics. Eur J Clin Invest 50(5):e13227
12. Amin S (2020) The psychology of coronavirus fear: are healthcare professionals suffering from corona-phobia? Int J Healthcare Manag 13(3):249–256
13. Seitz BM et al (2020) The pandemic exposes human nature: 10 evolutionary insights. Proc Natl Acad Sci 117(45):27767–27776
14. Zhang D (2021) Sinophobic epidemics in America: historical discontinuity in disease-related yellow peril imaginaries of the past and present. J Med Humanities 42(1):63–80
15. Belfi EL (2021) Examining the failure to care: shaming as a public health strategy during & beyond the coronavirus pandemic

16. Stuart H, Arboleda-Florez J, Sartorius N (2011) Paradigms lost: fighting stigma and the lessons learned. Oxford University Press
17. Ransing R et al (2020) Infectious disease outbreak related stigma and discrimination during the COVID-19 pandemic: drivers, facilitators, manifestations, and outcomes across the world. Brain Behav Immun 89:555
18. Van Bortel T et al (2016) Psychosocial effects of an Ebola outbreak at individual, community and international levels. Bull World Health Organ 94(3):210
19. de Melo-Martín I, Intemann K (2014) Who's afraid of dissent? Addressing concerns about undermining scientific consensus in public policy developments. Perspect Sci 22(4):593–615
20. Delborne JA (2015) Suppression and dissent in science. Handbook of academic integrity, pp 1–11
21. Crandall CS (2019) Science as dissent: the practical value of basic and applied science. J Soc Issues 75(2):630–641
22. Hamilton LC (2016) Public awareness of the scientific consensus on climate. SAGE Open 6 (4):2158244016676296
23. Landrum AR, Hallman WK, Jamieson KH (2019) Examining the impact of expert voices: communicating the scientific consensus on genetically-modified organisms. Environ Commun 13(1):51–70
24. De Regt HW (2017) Understanding scientific understanding. Oxford University Press
25. Spier R (2002) The history of the peer-review process. Trends Biotechnol 20(8):357–358
26. Ali PA, Watson R (2016) Peer review and the publication process. Nurs Open 3(4):193–202
27. Brezis ES, Birukou A (2020) Arbitrariness in the peer review process. Scientometrics 123 (1):393–411
28. Lewandowsky S, Gignac GE, Vaughan S (2013) The pivotal role of perceived scientific consensus in acceptance of science. Nat Clim Chang 3(4):399–404
29. Shwed U, Bearman PS (2010) The temporal structure of scientific consensus formation. Am Sociol Rev 75(6):817–840
30. Cook J (2016) Countering climate science denial and communicating scientific consensus. In: Oxford research encyclopedia of climate science
31. Kabat GC (2017) Taking distrust of science seriously: To overcome public distrust in science, scientists need to stop pretending that there is a scientific consensus on controversial issues when there is not. EMBO Rep 18(7):1052–1055
32. Maibach EW, van der Linden SL (2016) The importance of assessing and communicating scientific consensus. Environ Res Lett 11(9):091003
33. Conti K et al (2020) The evolving interplay between social media and international health security: a point of view. In: contemporary developments and perspectives in international health security, vol 1. IntechOpen
34. Stawicki SP, Firstenberg MS, Papadimos TJ (2020) The growing role of social media in international health security: the good, the bad, and the ugly. Global Health Security. Springer, pp 341–357
35. Papadimos TJ et al (2020) COVID-19 blind spots: a consensus statement on the importance of competent political leadership and the need for public health cognizance. J Global Infectious Diseases 12(4):167
36. Stawicki SP et al (2020) The 2019–2020 novel coronavirus (severe acute respiratory syndrome coronavirus 2) pandemic: a joint american college of academic international medicine-world academic council of emergency medicine multidisciplinary COVID-19 working group consensus paper. J Global Infectious Diseases 12(2):47
37. Trotter G (2021) COVID-19 and the authority of science. In: Hec Forum. Springer
38. Goldberg RF, Vandenberg LN (2021) The science of spin: targeted strategies to manufacture doubt with detrimental effects on environmental and public health. Environ Health 20(1):1–11
39. Kouzy R et al (2020) Coronavirus goes viral: quantifying the COVID-19 misinformation epidemic on Twitter. Cureus 12(3)

40. Trethewey SP (2019) Medical misinformation on social media: cognitive bias, Pseudo-Peer review, and the good intentions hypothesis. Circulation 140(14):1131–1133
41. Geoghegan S, O'Callaghan KP, Offit PA (2020) Vaccine safety: myths and misinformation. Front Microbiol 11:372
42. Carrieri V, Madio L, Principe F (2019) Vaccine hesitancy and (fake) news: quasi-experimental evidence from Italy. Health Econ 28(11):1377–1382
43. Chang LV (2018) Information, education, and health behaviors: Evidence from the MMR vaccine autism controversy. Health Econ 27(7):1043–1062
44. Smith MJ et al (2008) Media coverage of the measles-mumps-rubella vaccine and autism controversy and its relationship to MMR immunization rates in the United States. Pediatrics 121(4):e836–e843
45. Lynch A (2008) Thought contagion: how belief spreads through society: the new science of memes. Basic Books
46. Efferson C, McKay R, Fehr E (2020) The evolution of distorted beliefs vs. mistaken choices under asymmetric error costs. Evoluti Human Sci 2
47. Cataldi JR, Dempsey AF, O'Leary ST (2016) Measles, the media, and MMR: impact of the 2014–15 measles outbreak. Vaccine 34(50):6375–6380
48. Cacciatore MA, Nowak GJ, Evans NJ (2018) It's complicated: the 2014–2015 US measles outbreak and parents' vaccination beliefs, confidence, and intentions. Risk Anal 38(10):2178–2192
49. Zucker JR et al (2020) Consequences of undervaccination—measles outbreak, New York City, 2018–2019. N Engl J Med 382(11):1009–1017
50. Sanyaolu A et al (2019) Measles outbreak in unvaccinated and partially vaccinated children and adults in the United States and Canada (2018–2019): a narrative review of cases. INQUIRY J Health Care Organ Provision Financ 56:0046958019894098
51. Control CFD and Prevention (2019) US measles cases in first five months of 2019 surpass total cases per year for past 25 years. Press Release 30
52. Navar AM (2019) Fear-based medical misinformation and disease prevention: from vaccines to statins. JAMA cardiology 4(8):723–724
53. Burki T (2019) Vaccine misinformation and social media. Lancet Digital Health 1(6):e258–e259
54. Yeomans ND (2011) The ulcer sleuths: the search for the cause of peptic ulcers. J Gastroenterol Hepatol 26:35–41
55. Marshall B (2002) Helicobacter pioneers. Black-well Science Asia, Carlton, South Victoria ua
56. Thagard P (1997) Ulcers and bacteria I: discovery and acceptance
57. Thagard P (1997) Ulcers and bacteria II: Instruments, experiments, and social interactions
58. Fukuda Y et al (2001) The history of Helicobacter pylori. Rinsho byori. Jpn J Clin Pathol 49 (2):109–115
59. Konturek J (2003) Discovery by Jaworski of Helicobacter pylori. J Physiol Pharmacol 54 (S3):23–41
60. Mattila J (2016) The blockchain phenomenon–the disruptive potential of distributed consensus architectures. ETLA working papers
61. Sankar LS, Sindhu M, Sethumadhavan M (2017) Survey of consensus protocols on blockchain applications. In: 2017 4th international conference on advanced computing and communication systems (ICACCS). IEEE
62. Stawicki S, Firstenberg M, Papadimos T (2018) What's new in academic medicine? Blockchain technology in health-care: bigger, better, fairer, faster, and leaner. Int J Acad Med 4(1):1–11
63. Sunstein CR (2005) Why societies need dissent, vol 9. Harvard University Press
64. Jones PM (2017) Industry, enlightenment and dissent. In: Industrial enlightenment. Manchester University Press
65. Martin B (2014) Dissent in science

66. Hoffmann CH (2021) Making more research count: a blockchain enabled one-stop shop for immutable behavioral research. Foresight
67. Pritchard N (2021) Using blockchain technology to enable reproducible science
68. Hofmann F et al (2017) The immutability concept of blockchains and benefits of early standardization. In: 2017 ITU Kaleidoscope: challenges for a data-driven society (ITU K). IEEE
69. Puthal D et al (2018) The blockchain as a decentralized security framework [future directions]. IEEE Consumer Electron Mag 7(2):18–21
70. Rodriguez MA, Bollen J (2008) An algorithm to determine peer-reviewers. In: Proceedings of the 17th ACM conference on Information and knowledge management
71. D'Andrea R, O'Dwyer JP (2017) Can editors save peer review from peer reviewers? PLoS ONE 12(10):e0186111
72. Tenorio-Fornés A et al (2019) Towards a decentralized process for scientific publication and peer review using blockchain and IPFS. In: Proceedings of the 52nd Hawaii international conference on system sciences
73. van Rossum J (2018) The blockchain and its potential for science and academic publishing. Inf Serv Use 38(1–2):95–98
74. Dhillon V (2020) Blockchain based peer-review interfaces for digital medicine. Frontiers in Blockchain 3:8
75. Gupta DM, Boland RJ, Aron DC (2017) The physician's experience of changing clinical practice: a struggle to unlearn. Implement Sci 12(1):1–11
76. Manski CF (2010) Unlearning and discovery. Am Econ 55(1):9–18
77. Hanifatunnisa R, Rahardjo B (2017) Blockchain based e-voting recording system design. In: 2017 11th international conference on telecommunication systems services and applications (TSSA). IEEE
78. Koteska B, Karafiloski E, Mishev A (2017) Blockchain implementation quality challenges: a literature. In: SQAMIA 2017: 6th workshop of software quality, analysis, monitoring, improvement, and applications
79. Ismail L et al (2019) Towards a blockchain deployment at uae university: performance evaluation and blockchain taxonomy. In: Proceedings of the 2019 international conference on blockchain technology
80. Fan K et al (2018) Medblock: efficient and secure medical data sharing via blockchain. J Med Syst 42(8):1–11
81. Zhang G et al (2018) Blockchain-based data sharing system for ai-powered network operations. J Commun Inform Netw 3(3):1–8
82. Xia Q et al (2017) MeDShare: trust-less medical data sharing among cloud service providers via blockchain. IEEE Access 5:14757–14767
83. Tijdink JK, Verbeke R, Smulders YM (2014) Publication pressure and scientific misconduct in medical scientists. J Empir Res Hum Res Ethics 9(5):64–71
84. Gandevia S (2018) Publication pressure and scientific misconduct: why we need more open governance. 2018, Nature Publishing Group, pp 821–822
85. Fox MF (1994) Scientific misconduct and editorial and peer review processes. J Higher Educ 65(3):298–309
86. Misra DP, Agarwal V (2020) Blaming the peer reviewer: don't shoot the messenger!! Indian J Rheumatology 15(3):162
87. Baxt WG et al (1998) Who reviews the reviewers? Feasibility of using a fictitious manuscript to evaluate peer reviewer performance. Ann Emerg Med 32(3):310–317
88. Stawicki SP, Firstenberg MS, Papadimos TJ (2020) The growing role of social media in international health security: the good, the bad, and the ugly. Global Health Security, p 341
89. Le NK et al (2020) international health security: a summative assessment by acaim consensus group. In: Contemporary developments and perspectives in international health security, vol 1. IntechOpen

90. Mitchell A et al (2019) Many Americans say made-up news is a critical problem that needs to be fixed. Pew Research Center 5:2019
91. Common Program Requirements. Available from: https://www.acgme.org/what-we-do/accreditation/common-program-requirements/
92. Ahn J-W et al (2019) Blockchain for open scientific research. Google Patents

Index

© The Editor(s) (if applicable) and The Author(s), under exclusive license to Springer
Nature Switzerland AG 2023
S. Stawicki (ed.), *Blockchain in Healthcare*, Integrated Science 10,
https://doi.org/10.1007/978-3-031-14591-9

Printed in the United States
by Baker & Taylor Publisher Services